Sterile Products and Aseptic Techniques for the Pharmacy Technician

Mike Johnston, CPhT

Jeff Gricar, CPhT, M.Ed
Robin Luke, CPhT

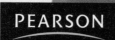

Boston   Columbus   Indianapolis   New York   San Francisco   Upper Saddle River
Amsterdam   Cape Town   Dubai   London   Madrid   Milan   Munich   Paris   Montreal   Toronto
Delhi   Mexico City   Sao Paulo   Sydney   Hong Kong   Seoul   Singapore   Taipei   Tokyo

Library of Congress Cataloging-in-Publication Data

Johnston, Mike, CPhT.
Sterile products and aseptic techniques for the pharmacy technician/Mike Johnston;
contributing authors, Jeff Gricar, Robin Luke.—2nd ed.
    p. ; cm.
Rev. ed. of: The pharmacy technician series. Sterile products. 2006.
Includes index.
ISBN-13: 978-0-13-510964-9
ISBN-10: 0-13-510964-7
1. Drugs—Sterilization.   2. Asepsis and antisepsis.   3. Pharmacy technicians.
I. Gricar, Jeff.   II. Luke, Robin.   III. Pharmacy technician series. Sterile products.   IV. Title.
    [DNLM: 1. Sterilization—methods.   2. Technology, Pharmaceutical—standards.
    3. Drug Compounding—standards.   4. Drug Contamination—prevention & control.
    5. Equipment and Supplies—standards.   6. Pharmacists' Aides. QV 778 J725s 2010]
RS199.S73J637 2010
615'.1076—dc22

2010025978

Publisher: Julie Levin Alexander
Publisher's Assistant: Regina Bruno
Editor-in-Chief: Mark Cohen
Executive Editor: John Goucher
Associate Editor: Bronwen Glowacki
Editorial Assistant: Mary Ellen Ruitenberg
Director of Marketing: David Gesell
Senior Marketing Manager: Katrin Beacom
Marketing Specialist: Michael Sirinides
Marketing Assistant: Judy Noh
Managing Production Editor: Patrick Walsh
Production Liaison: Julie Boddorf
Production Editor: Niraj Bhatt
Senior Media Editor: Amy Peltier

Media Project Manager: Lorena Cerisano
Manufacturing Manager: Ilene Sanford
Manufacturing Buyer: Pat Brown
Senior Art Director: Maria Guglielmo
Art Director: Christopher Weigand
Cover Designer: Kevin Kall
Cover Photo: Daniel Grill/Getty Images
Composition: Aptara®, Inc.
Printing and Binding: R.R. Donnelley/Willard
Cover Printer: Phoenix Color Corporation
The NPTA logo is a trademark of the National Pharmacy Technician
Association
The Straden-Schaden and RxPress logos are both trademarks of
Straden-Schaden, Inc.

Notice: The author and the publisher of this volume have taken care to make certain that the doses of drugs and schedules of treatment are correct and compatible with the standards generally accepted at the time of publication. Nevertheless, as new information becomes available, changes in treatment and in the use of drugs become necessary. The reader is advised to carefully consult the instruction and information material included in the package insert of each drug or therapeutic agent before administration. This advice is especially important when using, administering, or recommending new and infrequently used drugs. The author and publisher disclaim all responsibility for any liability, loss, injury, or damage incurred as a consequence, directly or indirectly, of the use and application of any of the contents of this volume. It is the responsibility of the reader to familiarize himself or herself with the policies and procedures set by the federal, state, and local agencies as well as the institution or agency where the reader may be employed. It is the reader's responsibility to stay informed of any new changes or recommendations made by any federal, state, and local agency as well as by his or her employing institution or agency.

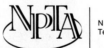

National Pharmacy
Technician Association

The NPTA logo is a trademark of the
National Pharmacy Technician Association

straden-schaden, inc.®

RxPRESS
PUBLICATIONS®

The Straden-Schaden and RxPress logos are
both trademarks of Straden-Schaden, Inc.

10 9 8 7 6 5 4

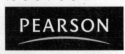

www.pearsonhighered.com

ISBN-13: 978-0-13-510964-9
ISBN-10:   0-13-510964-7

Dedication

To my grandparents . . . *You've built a strong, close, and admirable family— a rarity by today's standards. Our tree stands tall because of the roots held by you both. You demonstrated the meaning of hard work, good times, and the love that can be given only by a grandparent.*

"Nothing is so strong as gentleness, and nothing is so gentle as real strength."—Anonymous

Contents

PREFACE   vii

ABOUT THE AUTHORS   viii

ABOUT THE NATIONAL PHARMACY
TECHNICIAN ASSOCIATION   ix

ACKNOWLEDGMENTS   x

CONTRIBUTORS   xi

REVIEWERS   xii

chapter 1
Introduction to Sterile Products   1

Introduction   1

Parenteral Routes of Administration   2

Intravenous Infusions   3

Aseptic Technique   4

Sterile Products: Terminology and Abbreviations   4

    Conclusion   8
    Profiles of Practice   8
    Chapter Terms   8
    Chapter Review Questions   8

chapter 2
USP 797 Guidelines: Compounding Areas and Equipment   11

Introduction   11
    USP <797> Guidebook to Pharmaceutical Compounding—
        Sterile Preparations   12
    Facilities and Clean Room   13
    Clean Room   14
    Clean Air Space   14

Primary Engineering Controls   15
    Other Supplies   19

The Dressings (Garb)   19
    Personal Protection Equipment   19

Compounding Supplies   20
    Alcohol Pads   21
    Needles   21
    Syringes   21
    Miscellaneous   23
        Conclusion   27
        Profiles of Practice   27
        Chapter Terms   27
        Chapter Review Questions   27

chapter 3
Aseptic Calculations   30

Introduction   30

Intravenous Additive Dosage Calculations   31

Diluent, Powder, and Final Volume of
    Reconstituted Powder Vials   33

Milliequivalents   36

Intravenous Flow Rates   36

Intravenous Frequency or Schedule   37

Intravenous Drip Rates   37

Percentage Concentrations   39

Alligations   42

Electrolytes Added to Total Parenteral
    Nutrition Preparations   46

Dilution Technique   48
    Conclusion   48
    Chapter Review Questions   48

chapter 4
Properties of Sterile Products   53

Introduction   53

Particulate Matter   54

pH, Acids, and Bases   54
    The pH Scale   54

Compatibility and Stability   55
    Tonicity   56

Osmolality and Osmolarity   56
    Conclusion   57
    Chapter Terms   57
    Chapter Review Questions   57

chapter 5
Aseptic Technique   60

Introduction   60

Preparation   61
    Dressing   61
    Hand Washing   61

Proper Aseptic Technique   62
    Manipulation   63
    More on Manipulation   67
    Preparing a Sterile Dosage Form   72

Additional Aseptic Procedures 74
  Conclusion 75
  Profiles of Practice 75
  Chapter Terms 76
  Chapter Review Questions 76

chapter 6
Sterile Product Preparations 79

Introduction 79
Intravenous Bags 80
  Intravenous Piggybacks 80
  Continuous Preparations 81
Syringes 82
Multidose Vials 82
Patient-Controlled Analgesia 83
Epidurals 83
Neonates and Pediatric Patients 83
Irrigations 84
Cytotoxic Agents 84
Total Parenteral Nutrition 84
Proteins 84
  Albumin 84
  Plasma Protein Fraction 85
  Immunoglobulin 85
  Factor VIII 85
  Factor IX 86
Ophthalmics 86
  Conclusion 87
  Chapter Terms 87
  Chapter Review Questions 87

chapter 7
Total Parenteral Nutrition 89

Introduction 89
The Ingredients 90
  Fluid Maintenance 90
  Calories and Carbohydrates 90
  Amino Acids 91
  Electrolytes and Minerals 91
The Order 91
Compounding the Total Parenteral
  Nutrition 93
Automated Devices 95
  Automix 3+3 95
  Micromix 95

  Conclusion 96
  Profiles of Practice 96
  Chapter Terms 96
  Chapter Review Questions 96

chapter 8
Chemotherapy 99

Introduction 99
Cytotoxic Agents 101
Compounding Chemotherapy Medications 102
  Preparation Areas 102
  Personnel Training 108
  Attire 109
Procedures for Handling Sterile Injectable
  Hazardous Drugs 111
  PhaSeal 112
Disposal of Cytotoxic Medications 113
Chemotherapy Spills 113
ASHP Guidelines for Safe Handling of
  Cytotoxic Drugs 114
A Final Caution 115
  Conclusion 115
  Chapter Terms 115
  Chapter Review Questions 116

chapter 9
Quality Control and Assurance 118

Introduction 118
Elements of Quality in Pharmacy 119
  The Seven Rights 119
  Quality Assurance Functions 119
  Quality Improvement 119
Guidelines 120
  Food and Drug Administration 120
  The Joint Commission 120
  Centers for Disease Control and Prevention 120
  American Society of Health-System Pharmacists 120
  United States Pharmacopeia 121
  Miscellaneous 121
ASHP Guidelines on Quality Assurance for
  Pharmacy-Prepared Sterile Products 121
  Risk Level 1 121
  Risk Level 2 123
  Risk Level 3 125
United States Pharmacopeia 797 126
  Risk Levels 127
  Low-Risk-Level Compounded Sterile Products 127
  Medium-Risk-Level Compounded Sterile Products 128

High-Risk-Level Compounded Sterile Products   128
Environmental Sampling Testing   129
Cleaning and Disinfecting The Compounding Area   129
Policies and Procedures   130
Personnel, Education, and Evaluation   130
Storage and Handling inside and outside the Pharmacy   130
Facilities and Equipment   130
Aseptic Technique, Product Preparation, and Garb   130
Process Validation   130
End-Product Evaluation   131

Documentation and Labeling   131

Conclusion   132
Chapter Terms   132
Chapter Review Questions   132

APPENDICES

Appendix A: TERMINOLOGY AND ABBREVIATIONS   134
Appendix B: COMMON INTRAVENOUS MEDICATIONS   137
Appendix C: TRAINING AND VALIDATION FORMS   140
Appendix D: INSTRUCTIONS FOR LEFT-HANDED
          PERSONNEL   160
Appendix E: INSTITUTIONAL INTRAVENOUS
          CERTIFICATION TEST   166

INDEX   173

Preface

Sterile Products and Aseptic Techniques for the Pharmacy Technician is a core title in Pearson Education's pharmacy technician educational list of books. This text has been developed and designed to ensure greater success for the pharmacy technician student.

About the Book

Sterile product preparation and aseptic technique are advanced skills for pharmacy technicians. While this training provides extended career opportunities, these are challenging and precise skills to learn. This book, however, has been designed to guide the student through with ease, as each theory builds on those presented in earlier chapters.

The core features of this book include the following:

- Chapter introductions and summaries, which provide the student with a clearer understanding and rationale of the content being covered.

- Current, step-by-step instructions with color photographs of various aseptic techniques.

- Workplace Wisdom sections provide quick, highlighted tips and comments that replicate the advice of a seasoned intravenous technician.

- Profiles in Practice provide practical exercises that simulate real-world pharmacy problems or give students additional information and resources.

- Chapter review questions provide a learning assessment for both students and instructors to assess concept comprehension.

- Appendix B, Common Intravenous Medications, provides a current listing of common intravenous medications used in the United States. Drugs are categorized alphabetically by both generic name and trade name, and their use and classification are also provided.

- Appendix C, Training and Validation Forms, provides documentation that students and instructors can use with lab practicums, skills analysis, or even certification programs.

- Appendix D, Instructions for Left-Handed Personnel, should be of tremendous value for those who are left-handed or who train individuals who are. Left-handed trainees have been frustrated for years in trying to master aseptic technique, as all instructional material has been designed from a right-handed perspective. Step-by-step photos showing left-handed procedures have been included for all baseline aseptic techniques.

New to the Edition

In addition to enhancing and updating the original content, we have added:

- An Institutional Certification Practice Exam (Appendix E)

- An expanded and updated section explaining USP 797

- Lab activities to the end of each chapter to make this a worktext

- MyHealthProfessionsKit

About the Authors

Jeff Gricar, CPhT, M.Ed Jeff earned his pharmacy technician certificate in 1986 while serving in the U.S. Navy. He has extensive work experience in institutional, retail, and home health pharmacy settings. Pharmacy Technician Certification Board certified for more than 14 years, Jeff holds an undergraduate degree in business administration and a master's of education. As a full-time faculty member, he has taught and trained pharmacy technician students for Houston Community College's American Society of Health-System Pharmacists accredited Pharmacy Technician program since 1995. He is currently pursuing his doctorate degree.

Robin Luke, CPhT Robin is a founding member of the National Pharmacy Technician Association's Executive Advisory Board—the elected body of leaders for the association. She has more than 10 years of experience in institutional pharmacy, sterile product preparation, compounding, bulk manufacturing, and management, with a specialized knowledge of herbals and homeopathic treatments.

Robin has developed a variety of continuing-education programs with a strong emphasis on reducing medication errors; she also speaks at meetings and conferences across the United States.

with

Mike Johnston, CPhT Mike is known internationally as a respected author and speaker in the field of pharmacy. He published his first book, *Rx for Success—A Career Enhancement Guide for Pharmacy Technicians*, in 2002.

In 1999, Mike founded the National Pharmacy Technician Association in Houston, Texas, and led the association from 3 members to more than 20,000 in less than 2 years. Today, as executive director of the association and publisher of *Today's Technician* magazine, he spends the majority of his time meeting with and speaking to employers, manufacturers, association leaders, and elected officials on issues related to pharmacy technicians.

About the National Pharmacy Technician Association

The National Pharmacy Technician Association (NTPA) is the world's largest professional organization established specifically for pharmacy technicians. The association is dedicated to advancing the value of pharmacy technicians and the vital roles they play in pharmaceutical care. In a society of countless associations, we believe that it takes much more than a mission statement to meet the professional needs and provide the required leadership for the pharmacy technician profession—it takes action and results.

The organization is composed of pharmacy technicians practicing in a variety of practice settings, such as retail, independent, hospital, mail order, home care, long-term care, nuclear, military, correctional facility, formal education, training, management, and sales. NPTA is a reflection of this diverse profession and provides unparalleled support and resources to members.

NPTA is the foundation of the pharmacy technician profession; we have an unprecedented past, a strong presence, and a promising future. We are dedicated to improving our profession while remaining focused on our members.

For more information on NPTA:
Call 888-247-8700
Visit www.pharmacytechnician.org

Acknowledgments

Special Thanks to SaveWay Compounding Pharmacy

Bear, DE, Professional Compounding Centers of America (Houston, TX), and Clarian Health System (Indianapolis, IN) for your assistance with this text. Nearly every photograph in this book was shot on location at your facilities. I am grateful for the assistance, patience, and collaboration of your entire staff.

I would also like to thank Jeremy Van Pelt (photographer) and Multi Med Media (production management).

Jeff—Your revisions to the second edition have made this a better and stronger book. I appreciate your dedication to this project.

Bronwen—It has always been a pleasure working with you, and I am delighted to have had you manage the revisions to the second edition. You have done a simply amazing job.

Mark—Thank you for believing in my initial vision and concept for this series, which was anything but traditional. I will always remember the day we spent in New York City talking about cover concepts and the like at coffee shops and art galleries. More important, I am honored to have gotten to know you, Alex, and now little Sophie— and I consider each of you a friend.

Joan—You are truly gifted at what you do. I am amazed at your ability to join this project at the point you did and to guide each daunting task into a smooth and successful accomplishment. I feel that your leadership has created a better final product.

Julie—Thank you for taking risks (plural) on this project, compared with standard policies and procedures. In the end, your support and belief in this project have allowed a truly innovative product to be published.

Josh—Thank you for your detailed and comprehensive review of this project. Your commitment to accuracy and attention to detail have made this a better book.

Robin—Your commitment to this project—to exceeding all expectations, and to developing the best training series for pharmacy technicians available—has been amazing. You are a wonderful, gifted individual—but most important I am thankful to call you a friend.

Andrew and Jenny—Thank you supporting this project, each in your own unique ways; thank you for supporting me and the entire organization. This project tested each of us, our character, and our will, and I am honored to know you both.

Most important, I wish to thank my family. The last several years have been difficult and trying, but the strength, love, and support that you have given me have always pulled me through. *Thank you.*

Contributors

Jennifer Fix, RPh, MBA
Haltom City, TX

Linda F. McElhiney, PharmD, RPh
Clarian Health
Indianapolis, IN

Karen Orth, CPhT
Austin Community College
Austin, TX

Carol Reyes, CPhT
Oncology Specialists, S.C.
Franklin Park, IL

Reviewers

The reviewers of *Sterile Products and Aseptic Techniques for the Pharmacy Technician* have provided many excellent suggestions and ideas for improving this text. The quality of the reviews has been outstanding, and the reviews have been a major aid in the preparation of the manuscript. The assistance provided by these experts is deeply appreciated.

Lisa C. Barnes, BPharm, MBA
ACPE Program Administrator
University of Montana School of
Pharmacy and Allied Health Sciences
Missoula, MT

Roger B. Blair, MS, PAC, CPhT
Dean of Academics Virginia
College School of Business and
Health Chattanooga, TN

Kimberly Brown, AS, BUS, CPhT
Director and Instructor of Pharmacy
Technician Program Walters State
Community College Morristown, TN

Ralph P. Casas, PharmD, PhD
Associate Professor of Pharmacology
Cerritos Community College Norwalk, CA

Jane W. Dumas, MSN, CCMA, CHI
Allied Health Department Chair Remington
College–Cleveland West Campus North
Olmsted, OH

Kristie Fitzgerald, BSPharm
Clinical Pharmacist, Department of
Neonatology; Instructor Salt Lake
Community College Salt Lake City, UT

Michelle Goeking, BM, CPhT
Instructor Black Hawk College
Outreach Center Moline, IL

Madeline Jensen-Grauel, BSEd, MSci
Director, Pharmacy Technician
Training Program University of Texas
Medical Branch at Galveston Galveston, TX

Doris Klein, CMA, PT, BA
Medical Director Concorde Career
College San Diego, CA

Robert D. Kwiatkowski, BS, MA
Adjunct Instructor PIMA Medical
Institute Colorado Springs, CO

Tara Lynn Lebron CPhT
Clinical Coordinator/Lead
Instructor Sanford Brown
Institute Tampa, FL

Herminio Maldonado Jr, MS, BS
Pharmacy Technician Instructor PIMA
Medical Institute Colorado Springs, CO

Jennifer Meyers, CPhT
Lead Instructor, Pharmacy Technician
Program Virginia College at Austin Austin, TX

Bradley Moore, MSN
Director of Health Science Remington
Administrative Services Little Rock, AK

Hieu Nguyen, BS, CPhT
Pharmacy Technician Program
Director Western Career
College Sacramento, CA

And a special thank you to technical reviewer

Josh Cano, CPhT
Director of Education
National Pharmacy Technician Association

Introduction to Sterile Products

LEARNING OBJECTIVES

After completing this chapter, you should be able to:

- Define aseptic compounding and explain the need for sterile products.
- Distinguish and explain the various parenteral injection routes of administration.
- Explain why it is important that the parenteral administration route must be sterile or prepared aseptically.
- Describe the two mains type of venous access.
- Determine which types of parenteral administration must be preservative free.
- Describe the three methods of intravenous infusion.

Introduction

It is no longer necessary for most pharmacies to compound oral medications, unless alternative dosing or dosage forms are needed, as most medications dispensed today are manufactured by drug companies. However, many patients require intravenous therapy, in which case the pharmacy must compound the prescribed medications and solutions.

Pharmaceutical compounding is categorized as either nonsterile or sterile. Oral and topical mediations are commonly prepared with nonsterile compounding, while injections and intravenous admixtures are prepared by sterile compounding.

Intravenous therapy can be traced as far back as 1656, when Christopher Wren used a quill and bladder to inject opium into dogs; at that time, sterility did not play a factor. Fortunately, times have changed and so have the techniques for preparing and administering intravenous therapy.

Today, pharmacy technicians are in the forefront of preparing sterile products for administration to patients in both the institutional and home care settings by performing the majority of the sterile compounding in pharmacies. Therefore, it is imperative that technicians are properly trained and educated in regard to aseptic compounding and procedures to ensure that the compounded products remain sterile. Technicians who follow proper aseptic techniques and established guidelines will produce a sterile and contamination-free product for administration to the patient.

Workplace Wisdom

The word *aseptic* comes from the Latin prefix *a*, meaning "without," and the Latin word *sepsis*, meaning "infection." When using the term *aseptic*, we are talking about making or compounding a product without infection, also referred to as *sterile*.

Parenteral Routes of Administration

Parenteral routes of administration are used when a patient is unable to take medications by mouth, in emergency treatments when rapid absorption is essential, or when other dosage forms of the drug are not available. Injectable routes of administration are most commonly associated with the term *parenteral* and will be the focus of this text, but any route of administration that bypasses the gastrointestinal tract can be considered parenteral, such as transdermal and topical routes. Bypassing the gastrointestinal tract means that medications given via the parenteral route have a quicker onset of action than those given via most other routes of administration, and it is essential that any substance given via an injectable route be sterile.

The advantages of using an injectable route of administration are that there is a very rapid onset of action, drug levels can be more accurately controlled, it is good for irritant medications, and large volumes can be administered. However, there are disadvantages to an injectable route as well. First, this is the most dangerous route because once a drug is injected, it cannot be removed or retrieved from the body. In addition, it can be painful, and all the drugs must be prepared into an aqueous solution using aseptic technique.

Although there many different routes of **parenteral injection**, the pharmacy technician will most commonly prepare medications for intradermal, subcutaneous, intramuscular, and intravenous administration.

- **Intradermal (ID)**—an injection into the dermis or topmost layer of the skin. This route is most commonly used for skin tests for allergies and tuberculosis. Intradermal administration should not exceed volumes greater than 0.1 mL and should be administered using a small-gauge needle.

- **Subcutaneous (SC, SQ, subq)**—an injection into the fatty subcutaneous tissue of the skin. This route is used when slow and continuous absorption is required. For a smaller-gauge needle and with a maximum injection volume of 2 mL, common subcutaneous sites include the outer surface of the upper arms, the top of the thighs, the buttocks, and the abdomen. Because of the ease of administration and minimal pain and discomfort associated with this route, it is often used by patients for self-administration of drugs such as insulin, epinephrine, and low-molecular-weight heparin.

- **Intramuscular (IM)**—an injection deep into a large muscle mass, such as the buttocks, thighs, and upper arms. This is quicker acting than the subcutaneous route, and a maximum volume of 5 mL can be given IM, but any volume greater than 3 mL should be divided into two injections. The biggest disadvantage to IM injections is the pain that is normally associated with the injection.

- **Intravenous (IV)**—an injection directly into the bloodstream. This is the fastest option for parenteral administration because medication is introduced directly into the bloodstream. This is the preferred route for medications that are irritating, because they are quickly diluted. The IV route is not limited with regard to volume as are the other parenteral injection routes, but its use often is restricted by the patient's physical state. In general, an adult patient can receive more intravenous fluid than a pediatric or neonatal patient. In addition, a dehydrated patient can receive more intravenous fluid than a patient who is in congestive heart failure.

- **Intracardiac (IC)**—an injection directly into the cardiac muscle of the heart for emergency situations. Epinephrine is one of the most common IC medications and is available in a prefilled syringe with a 3½-in. needle, which allows for penetration through the chest wall.

- **Epidural**—an injection of medication or fluid directly into the epidural space or the space between the spinal cord and vertebrae. Epidurals can be used to treat neurologic pain and inflammation and commonly contain a narcotic drug and anesthetic such as bupivacaine or ropivacaine in a base solution of 0.9% sodium chloride or sterile water. It is very important to compound epidurals with preservative-free materials, as the presence of preservatives can cause permanent paralysis because preservatives cannot be broken down in the epidural space.

- **Intrathecal (IT)**—an injection of medication or fluid directly into the intrathecal space surrounding the spinal cord. This route is mainly used for spinal anesthesia, pain management, and chemotherapy. However, other drugs, such as baclofen, can be given intrathecally for the treatment of cerebral palsy. Like the epidural route, all intrathecal medication must be preservative free to prevent permanent paralysis or impaired cerebral function.

- **Intraperitoneal**—an injection directly into the peritoneal cavity or into an abdominal organ such as the kidney, liver, or bladder. It requires a 4- to 6-in. needle.

- **Intra-arterial (IA)**—an injection directly into an artery that leads to the desired organ of treatment. This route is typically used for diagnostic procedures but can also be used for chemotherapy medications.

- **Intraocular**—an injection directly into the eye. This is commonly used to treat ocular infections that do not respond to traditional treatment.

- **Intrapleural**—an injection directly into the pleural cavity. This is used to treat infections and cancers of the pleural cavity.

Intravenous Infusions

Intravenous infusions are administered through either a peripheral or a central vein. Access to these veins is made through a catheter or "line." Peripheral line access is made through veins located in the arms, legs, hands, and feet (Figure 1-1). Most commonly in a hospital setting, peripheral lines are meant to provide temporary venous access, as

Intravenous sites

Several sites on the body are used to intravenously administer drugs: the veins of the antecubital area (in front of the elbow), back of the hand, and some of the larger veins of the foot. On some occasions, a vein must be exposed by a surgical cut.

FIGURE 1-1 Intravenous administration sites

they can be dislodged easily. Peripheral lines need to be flushed on a regular basis with normal saline and/or heparin to clean the line and prevent blood coagulation. Commonly called heparin-lock flush, the heparin used to flush IV lines is in a very low concentration (10–100 units/mL) and dose (30–300 units per flush). Most intravenous medications compounded by a pharmacy technician will be infused via a peripheral line.

Central line access is made through veins in the neck (jugular) or chest (subclavian) or via peripheral insertion through the arm into the superior vena cava, the body's "central" or main vein. Central lines are used for various reasons. Central lines are used not only when peripheral access is not available and for long-term medication administration, but also to administer caustic substances (chemotherapy) and highly concentrated total parenteral nutrition (TPN). The central veins have more blood volume running through them than the peripheral veins, which allows the more caustic and concentrated medications to be administered without damaging the blood vessels.

Intravenous infusions can be categorized as an intravenous push, a continuous infusion, or an intermittent infusion. An **intravenous push (IVP)** is a small-volume injection (10 mL or less) directly from a syringe into the vein. A **continuous infusion** is a larger volume of solution (250 mL or more) infused at a constant rate over a longer administration time. An intermittent infusion or intravenous **piggyback** (IVPB) is a smaller volume of fluid (less than 250 mL) that is given at scheduled intervals and infused over a short period of time (usually less than 1 hours). Intermittent infusions are "piggybacked" into the continuous IV catheter to further dilute the medication and reduce irritation.

Aseptic Technique

Any medication or solution that is administered by parenteral injection must be sterile or free of any contamination, such as bacteria, **pyrogens**, and particulate matter. Utilizing proper aseptic technique is the only way that technicians can ensure that the products they prepare are sterile. Aseptic technique and methods are used to maintain the sterility of compounded products. Aseptic technique includes proper hygiene, garb, equipment, manipulations, and procedures, all of which are discussed in later chapters. If proper aseptic technique is not used in the preparation of sterile products, then the contamination in the product can be transferred directly into the patient's body, which in most cases is already compromised, causing serious health complications such as **phlebitis**, **sepsis**, or death.

Sterile Products: Terminology and Abbreviations

In order to be successful, the pharmacy technician preparing sterile products must fully understand not only the procedures, but also the terminology and abbreviations used in sterile compounding. Tables 1-1 to 1-4 give common terms and abbreviations that might be encountered by a pharmacy technician engaged in sterile compounding.

Table 1-1   Sterile Products Terminology

TERM	DEFINITION
Additive	Any drug or component added to an IV solution
Admixture	An IV solution with at least one medication added to it
Aerosolization	The spraying of small liquid or powder particles in the air; usually occurs when withdrawing a needle from a vial or when removing air from a syringe
Ampule	A sealed glass container containing sterile injectable medication
Bacteriocidal	An agent capable of killing bacteria

TERM	DEFINITION
Bacteriostatic	An agent capable of inhibiting the growth of bacteria
Bolus	An initial dose of medication or solution; usually a dose higher than the maintenance dose; also called loading dose
Central line	An IV access site into one of the major blood vessels; this is the IV line through which hypertonic fluids may be given
Compatibility	The ability of two or more components to be mixed together without physical or chemical degradation of any component
Contamination	The presence of a harmful or unwanted substance
Continuous infusion	An infusion given at a continuous rate over a long period of time
Coring	The breaking off of a part of the rubber stopper of a vial or container due to an improper needle stick; the cored part of the rubber stopper is usually pushed into the vial or container.
Critical site	Any opening or pathway that is at risk for contact with air or touch contamination
Diluent	The liquid used to reconstitute a powder drug or the liquid added to reduce the concentration of another liquid
Extravasation	A caustic or hazardous IV solution that has been inadvertently infused into the tissue surrounding the injection site
Infiltration	An IV solution that is inadvertently infused into the tissue surrounding the injection site
Infusion	The slow administration of mediation or solution via a parenteral route of administration
Intermittent infusion	An infusion given over specific and shorter periods of time
Intravenous piggyback	Delivery of a secondary IV solution into an existing IV line
Loading dose	An initial dose of a drug that is used to achieve a desired drug level
Multiple-dose vial	A vial that is intended for multiple needle punctures and withdrawals; usually contains preservatives to maintain sterility
Parenteral	Administration of a drug via a route of administration that bypasses the gastrointestinal tract (i.e., injection)
Particulate	Foreign objects or matter
Pathogen	Disease-causing organisms such as bacteria, fungus, and viruses
Peripheral line	An IV access site made through veins located in the arms, legs, hands, or feet
Preservative	Any additive intended to extend the content, stability, or sterility of a medication or solution
Pyrogen	Fever-producing organism
Reconstitution	Adding a diluent to a powder to create a liquid
Single-dose vial	A vial that contains no preservatives and is intended to be used only one time; not designed to maintain sterility after multiple puncture
Sterile compounding	The aseptic mixing of ingredients to prepare sterile medications (usually injectable) for patient use
Vial	A small glass or plastic container that holds injectable medications and solutions

Table 1-2   Intravenous Solution Abbreviations

ABBREVIATION	SOLUTION
¼ NS	¼ Normal saline: 0.225% sodium chloride
½ NS	½ Normal saline: 0.45% sodium chloride
D10W	Dextrose 10% in water
D20W	Dextrose 20% in water
D30W	Dextrose 30% in water
D5 ¼ NS	Dextrose 5% in ¼ normal saline
D5 ½ NS	Dextrose 5% in ½ normal saline
D50W	Dextrose 50% in water
D5LR	Dextrose 5% in Lactated Ringer's
D5NS	Dextrose 5% in normal saline
D5W	Dextrose 5% in water
D70W	Dextrose 70% in water
LR	Lactated Ringer's
NS	Normal saline; 0.9% sodium chloride

Table 1-3   Chemical Abbreviations

ABBREVIATION	SUBSTANCE
AHF	Antihemolytic factor (factor VIII, factor IX)
B_1	Vitamin B_1, thiamine
B_{12}	Vitamin B_{12}, cyanocobalamin
B_6	Vitamin B_6, pyridoxine
Ca	Calcium
Cl	Chloride
Cu	Copper
epi	Epinephrine
IgG	Immunoglobulin G
IVIG	Intravenous immune globulin
K	Potassium
K_3PO_4	Potassium phosphate
KCl	Potassium chloride
Mg	Magnesium
$MgSO_4$	Magnesium phosphate
MVI	Multivitamin injection
Na	Sodium
NaCl	Sodium chloride
$NaHCO_3$	Sodium bicarbonate
$NaPO_4$	Sodium phosphate
NTG	Nitroglycerin

ABBREVIATION	SUBSTANCE
PCN	Penicillin
PO_4	Phosphate
SO_4	Sulfate
SWFI	Sterile water for injection or sterile water for irrigation
TPA	Tissue plasminogen activator
Zn	Zinc

Table 1-4 Other Sterile Products Abbreviations

ABBREVIATION	STERILE PRODUCT
ACD	Automated compounding device
amp	Ampule
BSC	Biological safety cabinet
BUD	Beyond-use date
CACI	Compounding aseptic containment isolator
CAI	Compounding aseptic isolator
CSP	Compounded sterile product
DCA	Direct compounding area
G	Gauge
HEPA	High-efficiency particulate air filter
IA	Intra-arterial
IC	Intracardiac
ID	Intradermal
IM	Intramuscular
IPA	Isopropyl alcohol
ISO	International Organization for Standardization
IT	Intrathecal
IV	Intravenous
IVFE	Intravenous fat emulsion
IVP	Intravenous push
IVPB	Intravenous piggyback
KVO	Keep vein open
LAFW	Laminar airflow workbench
LAH	Laminar airflow hood
MDV	Multiple-dose vial, multidose vial
PCA	Patient-controlled analgesia
PEC	Primary engineering control
PF	Preservative free
PFS	Prefilled syringe

(continued)

Table 1-4   *(continued)*

ABBREVIATION	STERILE PRODUCT
PPE	Personnel protective equipment
PPN	Partial parenteral nutrition
SDV	Single-dose vial
SC, SQ, subq	Subcutaneous
SW	Sterile water
SWFI	Sterile water for injection or sterile water for irrigation
TKO	To keep vein open
TNA	Total nutrient admixture, a combination of TPN and IVFE
TPN	Total parenteral nutrition

CONCLUSION

Sterile products are a vital component of modern pharmaceutical care. Therefore, it is vital for pharmacy technicians to have a solid understanding and working knowledge of proper aseptic technique. Guidelines have been established for aseptic technique for the protection of both the patient and the personnel involved.

PROFILES OF PRACTICE

Depending on the state in which they practice, pharmacy technicians may compound most, if not all, sterile products. The roles of pharmacists are becoming increasingly clinical based: checking for possible allergies, duplicate orders, and correct dosages; serving as a reference for physicians and nurses; and many other clinical applications. With these increases in job responsibilities, the pharmacist needs help, and more pharmacy technicians are receiving training and attending classes to learn about aseptic techniques and compounding practices.

States that require pharmacy technicians to be certified and/or require that technicians register with the state board of pharmacy usually give technicians more responsibility. In some progressive states, pharmacy technicians may compound any type of sterile product, including intravenous admixtures, ophthalmic medications, total parenteral nutrition bags, and chemotherapy medications, all under the pharmacist's supervision, practicing what is universally known as aseptic technique.

CHAPTER TERMS

continuous infusion larger volume of solution (250 mL or more) infused at a constant rate over a longer administration time

intravenous push (IVP) small-volume injection (10 mL or less) directly from a syringe into the vein

parenteral injection administration via injection

phlebitis inflammation of a vein

piggyback (IVPB) delivery of a secondary IV solution from an outside source into an IV line containing fluid from an existing line

pyrogen a substance that produces fever

sepsis the presence of organisms in the blood

CHAPTER REVIEW QUESTIONS

MATCHING

Choose the correct description for the parenteral injection route.

1. ___e___ injection directly into muscle
2. ___d___ injection into the uppermost skin layer
3. ___f___ injection directly into the eye
4. ___b___ injection directly into the liver
5. ___c___ injection directly into the heart
6. ___a___ injection into the space between the spinal cord and vertebrae

a. epidural
b. intra-arterial
c. intracardiac
d. intradermal
e. intramuscular
f. intraocular

7. __K__ injection into the fatty layer of the skin
8. __j__ injection directly into a vein
9. __g__ injection directly into an artery
10. __h__ injection into the pleural cavity
11. __i__ injection into the space surrounding the spinal cord

g. intraperitoneal
h. intrapleural
i. intrathecal
j. intravenous
k. subcutaneous

Match the following abbreviations:

12. __c__ intradermal
13. __i__ total parenteral nutrition
14. __g__ intravenous push
15. __a__ intravenous
16. __d__ immunoglobulin G
17. __e__ intramuscular
18. __b__ patient-controlled analgesia
19. __f__ intravenous immune globulin
20. __h__ intravenous piggyback

a. IV
b. PCA
c. ID
d. IgG
e. IM
f. IVIG
g. IVP
h. IVPB
i. TPN

LAB ACTIVITIES

Transcribe the following abbreviations:

LAFW : _Laminar airflow workbench_
PEC: _Primary engineering control_
D5 ½ NS: _Dextrose 5% in normal saline_
$NaPO_4$: _Sodium phosphate_
BSC: _Biological Safety Cabinet_
D5W: _Dextrose 5% in Water_
HEPA: _High-efficiency particulate air filter_
NS: _Normal Saline / 9% Sodium chloride_
PPE: _Personnel protective equipment_
CAI: _Compounding aseptic isolater_
MDV: _Multiple Dose Vial - multidose vial_
IM: _Intramuscular_
DCA: _Direct Compounding area_
IVPB: _Intravenous piggybag_
SWFI: _Sterile water for injection_
IPA _Isopropyl alcohol_

D5LR: _Dextrose 5% in Lactated Ringers_
IVIG: _Intravenous immune globulin_
TPN: _Total parental Nutrition_
K_3PO_4: _Photassium Phosphate_
MVI: _Multivitamin injection_
IVFE: _Intravenous fat emulsion_
TKO: _To keep vein open_
PFS: _Prefilled syringe_
IV: _Intravenous_
PF: _Preservative free_
SDV: _Single dose vial_
BUD: _Beyond use date_
ACD: _Automated Compounding device_
D5 ¼ NS: _Dextrose 5% in normal Saline_
½ NS: _½ Normal saline_
D70W: _Dextrose 70% in Water_

Transcribe the following IV orders:

1. D5 ½ NS with 20 mEq KCl/L @ 80 mL/hr
Dextrose 0.5% in ½ normal Saline with 20 miliEquivalent Potassium Chloride

2. PCN 1,000,000 units IVPB q6h
Penicilin 1,000,000 units intravenous piggybag every 6 hours.

3. NS 500 mL with heparin 20,000 units @ 2000 units/hr
Normal saline 500 ml with heparin 20,000 units @ 2000 units per hour.

4. ½ NS 1 L with 1 g $MgSO_4$
½ normal saline 1 L with 1 g magnesium phosphate

5. B$_{12}$ 1000 mcg IM q week

Vitamin B12 1000 mcg
Intramuscular every week

6. Add B$_1$ 100 mg qd to TPN

Agregar Vitamin B, 100 mg
every day to Total Parenteral
nutrition

7. Prepare 1 L of 70% IPA

Prepare 1 L of 70%
Isopropyl alcohol

8. NTG 50 mg in 250 mL D5W infuse at 10 mcg/min

Nitroglicerin 50 mg in
250 ml Dextrose 5% in
Water infuse at 10 mcg per
minute

USP 797 Guidelines: Compounding Areas and Equipment

LEARNING OBJECTIVES

After completing this chapter, you should be able to:

- Explain the purpose of USP 797.
- Describe the difference among classes of ISO air environments.
- Explain the importance of aseptic technique in compounding.
- Describe the difference between an ante area and a buffer area.
- Define primary engineering control and give at least three examples.
- Define needle and syringe and which parts of each must remain sterile.

Introduction

Sterile compounding is used to prepare intravenous products, ophthalmics, and irrigations. The final product must be free from chemical and physical contaminants, accurately and correctly compounded, pharmaceutically elegant, pyrogen free, and stable for its intended shelf life. It must also be packaged in a manner that will ensure maintenance of its quality until it is used.

The area in which the compounding takes place is commonly referred to as a clean room or compounding area. The equipment used within the compounding area differs from facility to facility. There are, however, universal standards regarding facilities, equipment, and dress. These mandatory requirements and guidelines are set forth in the U.S. Pharmacopeia's (USP) *USP <797>Guidebook to Pharmaceutical Compounding—Sterile Preparations* (USP 797). Each facility should have a more specific policy pertaining to its needs in addition to these universal guidelines.

Whatever the practice setting in which the pharmacy technician spends his or her career, it will require some form of clothing specific to the company. For preparing sterile products, however, the items that the pharmacy technician will be required to wear may include various types of coverings for the face, eyes, hands, feet, and other body parts.

Four key factors contribute to the preparation of high-quality sterile products: facilities, environmental control, components, and operators.

USP <797> Guidebook to Pharmaceutical Compounding—Sterile Preparations

In January 2004, the USP issued a set of new and stringent regulations regarding aseptic preparations in USP 797. It includes a new approach to facility design, microbial contamination risk levels, personnel training and evaluation, clean room atmosphere, proper dress, quality assurance, validation, and monitoring. The purpose is "to prevent harm and death to patients treated with" compounded sterile products (CSPs). It deals with the preparation, storage, and transportation of compounded sterile products but does not discuss administration of those products. Previously, facilities operated under guidelines already set forth the by the USP and the American Society of Health-System Pharmacists. However, USP 797 expands on many of those previous criteria and sets the federal standard for facilities that compound sterile products. These guidelines became official on June 1, 2008.

Because IVs go directly into a patient's vein, there is no room for error, and they must be sterile and prepared under strict USP 797 guidelines. These guidelines were put in place to prevent harm or death from contamination, differences in component strengths, contaminants, and inappropriate quality of ingredients. USP 797 includes guidelines on the following:

- **Responsibility of Compounding Personnel**—This section discusses the responsibilities to ensure that the sterile products are compounded, labeled, stored, and dispensed properly.

- **CSP Microbial Contamination Risk Factors**—On the basis of their potential for contamination, this section categorizes compounded products into low-, medium-, or high-risk compounded sterile products and discusses each risk level in detail.

- **Personnel Training and Evaluation in Aseptic Manipulation Skills**—This section gives specific guidelines that personnel should follow to produce a sterile final product.

- **Immediate-Use CSPs**—This section details how to handle compounded products that are intended to be used immediately or in emergency situations.

- **Single-Dose and Multiple-Dose Containers**—This section defines the differences between a single- and multiple-dose container, including expiration dates and time frames.

- **Hazardous Drugs as CSPs, Radiopharmaceuticals as CSPs, and Allergen Extracts as CSPs**—This section details how these special types of compounded products should be handled.

- **Verification of Compounding Accuracy and Sterility**—This section discusses in detail the monitoring, testing, and documentation needed to ensure a sterile product.

- **Elements of Quality Control**—This section discusses how specific training and evaluations programs must be developed for all personnel involved in the compounding of sterile products.

- **Finished Preparation Release Checks and Tests**—This section details what types of testing and checks must be performed before a compounded sterile product is dispensed or administered to a patient.

- **Storage and Beyond-Use Dating**—This section details the requirements for storage and expiration dating of compounded sterile products.

- **Maintaining Sterility, Purity, and Stability of Dispensed and Distributed CSPs**—This section discusses how personnel and facilities can maintain the sterility, purity, and stability of compounded sterile products during packaging, handling, transportation, use, and storage.

- **Patient or Caregiver Training**—This section details how patients and caregivers should be trained to administer their own compounded sterile products.

- **Patient Monitoring and Adverse Events Reporting**—This section discusses how to monitor and report adverse drug reactions.

- **Quality Assurance (QA) Program**—This section discusses the characteristics of a compounded sterile product quality assurance plan.

Facilities and Clean Room

Facilities that perform aseptic sterile compounding must have a designated area for this task. This area should be placed in a section of the facility where traffic is very limited and airflow is unrestricted. Only designated personnel should enter this space and only for the purpose of aseptic preparations. The sterile compounding area should be large enough to accommodate necessary equipment, such as the primary engineering controls (PECs), and to provide for the proper storage of drugs and supplies under appropriate conditions of temperature, light, moisture, sanitation, ventilation, and security. Sterile compounding areas are Com rooms in which the air quality, temperature, and humidity are highly regulated in order to greatly reduce the risk of cross-contamination. The air in a clean room is repeatedly filtered to remove dust particles, **particulates**, and other impurities.

Workplace Wisdom

The environmental control of air is of concern because room air may be highly contaminated. For example, sneezing produces 100,000–200,000 aerosol droplets that can then attach to dust particles. These contaminated particles may be present in the air for weeks.

Air environments are now classified into six International Organization for Standardization (ISO) categories (formerly Federal Standard No. 209E [FS209E]). Air environments are rated as follows:

- ISO Class 3: contains no more than 35.2 particles of 0.5 micron or larger per cubic meter. An ISO 3 environment is equivalent to FS209E Class 1 (no more than 1 particle of 0.5 micron or larger per cubic foot).

- ISO Class 4: contains no more than 352 particles of 0.5 micron or larger per cubic meter. An ISO 4 environment is equivalent to FS209E Class 10 (no more than 10 particles of 0.5 micron or larger per cubic foot).

- ISO Class 5: contains no more than 3520 particles of 0.5 micron or larger per cubic meter. An ISO 5 environment is equivalent to FS209E Class 100 (no more than 100 particles of 0.5 micron or larger per cubic foot).

- ISO Class 6: contains no more than 35,200 particles of 0.5 micron or larger per cubic meter. An ISO 6 environment is equivalent to FS209E Class 1000 (no more than 1000 particles of 0.5 micron or larger per cubic foot).

- ISO Class 7: contains no more than 352,000 particles of 0.5 micron or larger per cubic meter. An ISO 7 environment is equivalent to FS209E Class 10,000 (no more than 10,000 particles of 0.5 micron or larger per cubic foot).

- ISO Class 8: contains no more than 3,520,000 particles of 0.5 micron or larger per cubic meter. An ISO 7 environment is equivalent to FS209E Class 100,000 (no more than 100,000 particles of 0.5 micron or larger per cubic foot).

Clean Room

USP 797 divides clean rooms or compounding areas into two distinct areas. The ante area or **anteroom** is an ISO Class 8 or better area where the compounding personnel perform aseptic hand washing and dressing procedures. Technicians also gather all necessary ingredients and supplies and perform order entry and labeling within the anteroom. The buffer area is the area in which the PEC is located. Buffer areas should be an ISO 7 or better environment. If the ante area and buffer area are not separate rooms, then there must be some type of demarcation that separates the two areas. The PEC is a device (LAFW, BSC, CAI, CACI) or room that maintains ISO 5 conditions for aseptic preparations. The direct compounding area (DCA) is the critical area within the ISO 5 PEC where aseptic manipulations are performed.

Access to the aseptic compounding areas should be limited to essential personnel only. No personnel should be allowed to approach the buffer area unless properly gowned, adequately trained, and validated. It is necessary to avoid horseplay or excessive movement near the hood, as this will disturb airflow.

Doors to the compounding area room must remain closed at all times. No food, drinks, or gum is allowed in the compounding area. Personnel should avoid coughing, sneezing, singing, whistling, or excessive talking while in compounding areas because this may also contribute to adding contaminants to the air. In addition, activities such as these can distract personnel, causing lost concentration and increasing the risk of medication errors.

All supplies should be externally clean and sanitized before they are brought into the buffer area. Within the anteroom area they are uncartoned, cleaned, and sanitized and then transferred to a clean cart restricted to the buffer area.

A further transfer barrier step should occur as supply items are introduced into the PEC. Whenever possible, external wrappings (such as IV outer bags and syringe pouches) should be removed at the edge of the PEC and supply items introduced into the PEC should be limited to those required for the planned procedure, and they should be arranged so as not to obstruct the HEPA airflow pattern and to provide for efficient processing.

Clean Air Space

The technician must perform all compounding at least 6 in. inside the edges of the PEC; this area is known as the clean air space. As the sterile air hits the sides of the PEC, the air is considered contaminated and no longer clean. As the air moves toward the outer edge of the hood, the room air begins to mix with the clean air, reducing sterility.

Just as the technician has appropriately prepared, the PEC must also be prepared. The blower should remain on at all times. If it has been turned off, it must be turned on for at least 30 minutes prior to use. The PEC must be cleaned with sterile water and 70% isopropyl alcohol or another sanitizing agent using a lint-free wipe or gauze.

The sterile compounding area must be segregated from other areas of the pharmacy and will have only one door, which should remain closed when not in use. It is a positive-pressure room, which means that when the door is opened, air will flow out of the area. It is designed to keep particulates from flowing into the room when the door is in use (Figure 2-1).

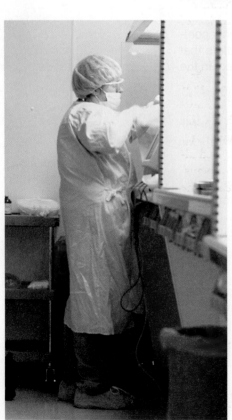

FIGURE 2-1 Clean room

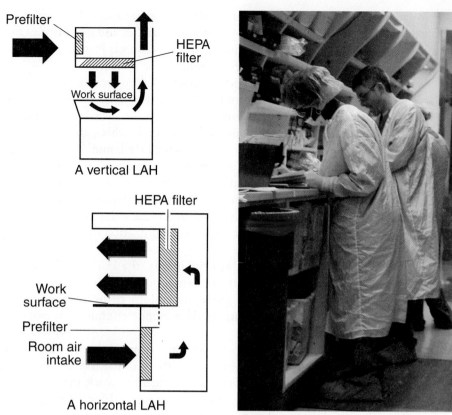

Prefilter

HEPA filter

Work surface

A vertical LAH

HEPA filter

Work surface

Prefilter

Room air intake

A horizontal LAH

FIGURE 2-2 Positive Pressure airflow

FIGURE 2-3 Anteroom

The purpose of the positive pressure is to keep unfiltered or dirty air from entering the clean room where the clean air is. The air in a clean room is purified so that it is cleaner than the air in the rest of the pharmacy and/or hospital. The cleaner the air, the less is the chance that contaminants will be introduced into a sterile product (Figure 2-2).

Only the supplies necessary for scheduled aseptic preparation, such as syringes, needles, and alcohol swabs, should be brought into the buffer area. The buffer area is not designed to store excessive amounts of supplies. The USP 797 states that "the surfaces of ceilings, walls, floors, fixtures, shelving, counters, and cabinets in the buffer area shall be smooth, impervious, free from cracks and crevices, and non-shedding." This will minimize contaminant, microorganisms, and dirt from accumulating and allows for ease when cleaning (Figure 2-3). Junctures of ceilings to walls, walls to walls, and floors to walls should be covered or caulked to make them easier to clean. The areas should have no dust-collecting ledges, pipes, or similar surfaces. Work surfaces should be durable and smooth and made of stainless steel or molded plastic. Carts should be of stainless steel wire or sheet construction with good-quality, cleanable casters and should be restricted to the controlled area.

Primary Engineering Controls

The USP 797 defines a primary engineering control as "a device or room that provides an ISO Class 5 environment for the exposure of critical sites when compounding" sterile products. PECs include laminar airflow workbenches (LAFWs), biological safety cabinets (BSCs), compounding aseptic isolators (CAIs), and compounding aseptic containment isolators (CACIs).

In the 1960s, due to the increased need for clean air in the industry, laminar airflow hoods (also known as *clean benches* or *laminar flow cabinets*) were first developed

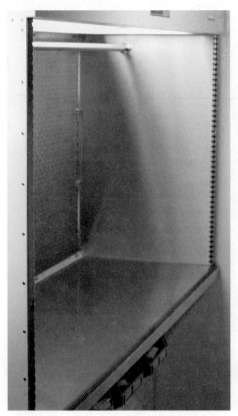

FIGURE 2-4 Laminar airflow hood

to provide product protection for small-scale experimental procedures. Today, laminar airflow hoods are used in most facilities and laboratories for all types of sterile product preparations and procedures. Pharmacy technicians work with airflow hoods to compound sterile products.

A laminar airflow hood provides a controlled environment in which levels of particulates, microbes, and contaminants of all kinds are regulated and kept to a minimum by constant air filtration. The hood creates a particle-free working environment by taking in air through a filtration system and exhausting it across a work surface in a laminar or unidirectional airstream. Commonly, the filtration system consists of a prefilter and a high-efficiency particulate air (HEPA) filter. Because the air within the cabinet does not contain any airborne particles (Figure 2-3), it is also sterile. The airflow hood is usually enclosed on the sides and kept under constant positive pressure in order to prevent infiltration of contaminated room air.

There are two main types of airflow hoods, the horizontal laminar airflow hood (LAFW) and the vertical airflow hood, or biological safety cabinet (BSC), and two types of glovebox isolators, the compounding aseptic isolator (CAI) and the compounding aseptic containment isolator (CACI).

The airflow in the LAFW flows horizontally from the back of the hood toward the front of the hood, whereas the airflow in the BSC flows vertically downward from the top of the hood toward the work surface. Each hood is designed to sterilize through filtration using a HEPA filter.

The function of airflow hoods is twofold:

- To filter bacteria and other particulate matter from the air
- To maintain a constant airflow out of the hood to prevent entry of contaminants.

Horizontal Laminar Airflow Hood

Most nonhazardous aseptic compounding should take place in the LAFW (Figure 2-4). The LAFW has a prefilter in the front or on top of the hood that removes any large contaminants from the room air. The prefilter should be changed monthly and documented. After the air has been filtered once through the prefilter, it travels to the back of the hood, where it is filtered again in the HEPA filter. The HEPA filter removes particles that are 0.2 micron and larger. That covers almost all bacteria, fungi, and viruses. The filtered air is then blown horizontally toward the front of the hood. The HEPA filter is not changed but should be tested every 6 months for efficiency. The LAFW must be turned on for at least 30 minutes before any aseptic compounding can take place.

Biological Safety Cabinet

Hazardous compounding (chemotherapy) takes place in the BSC (Figure 2-5). There are two main types of BSC, which differ based on where the filtered air from the BSC is exhausted. Both hoods have four sides with an 8- to 12-in. opening in the front. A sliding glass front can be brought down to the proper opening level.

The opening in the front allows the room air to be sucked into the BSC grills, which are located in the front and back of the inside of the hood's work surface area. This air is then filtered and circulated to the HEPA filter, which then filters the air to 0.3 micron. The filtered air is blown from the top of the hood vertically downward to the work surface area. The air is

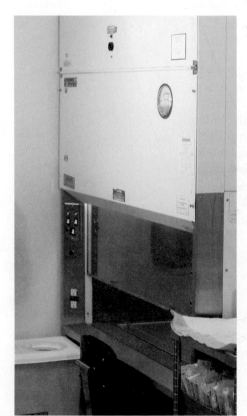

FIGURE 2-5 Biological safety cabinet

then filtered again and either eliminated back into the room air or to an outside vent. As with the LAH, the HEPA filter should be tested every 6 months.

Glovebox Isolator

The two types of glovebox isolators (CAI and CACI) can be used in lieu of having a clean room that meets USP 797 guidelines. Both isolators are self-contained environments where the operator manipulates the sterile products through the use of a glove system. The operator introduces the supplies necessary to compound the sterile product into the isolator's transfer chamber. After closing the transfer chamber door, the operator then inserts his or her hands into the isolator's gloves and opens the transfer chamber from inside the isolator to introduce the supplies into the work environment. After compounding, the operator places the CSP back into the transfer chamber and closes the inside door. The operator then removes his or her hands from the isolator's gloves and opens the outside transfer chamber door to remove the CSP.

The CAI uses positive pressure to ensure product and personnel protection and is used for nonhazardous sterile compounding. The CACI uses negative pressure to protect the product and personnel and is used for the compounding of hazardous CSPs. Both the CAI and CACI provide an ISO 5 environment for the preparation of sterile products and can contain two, three, or four glove ports.

Bacteria and surface contamination can be expected, even if it is not visible. Written standard procedures should be developed and followed for cleaning and sanitizing all surfaces within the controlled area. As mentioned previously, water and sterile 70% isopropyl alcohol or other **germicidal** products are typically used. All reusable cleaning tools, such as mops, should be restricted to the controlled area and thoroughly cleaned and sanitized after each use.

USP 797 requires that PECs be frequently and thoroughly cleaned and disinfected. Cleaning and disinfecting should occur, at a minimum, at the beginning of every shift, before the beginning of a batch compound, and every 30 minutes during continuous compounding of sterile products. PEC should also be cleaned when the surface is dirty or contaminated or if there are any spills. A compounder should wipe down the surface area when he or she is finished preparing one type of product and before compounding another. For example, when finished preparing a penicillin-based product, the compounder should wipe down the hood before mixing another product. This is because some patients may be allergic to penicillin, and in aseptic compounding one goal is to prevent cross-contaminants from entering a product.

PROCEDURE **2-1**

Cleaning the Hood

The technician should always clean the horizontal laminar airflow workbench from top to bottom, from the back to the front opening. The procedure for properly cleaning the hood is as follows (Figure 2-6):

1. Wash the entire hood walls and surface with sterile water to remove salt, starch, sugar, and/or proteins.
2. Soak stubborn spots for 5–10 minutes, then wipe clean.
3. To disinfect, wipe all the surfaces of the hood with sterile 70% isopropyl alcohol using lint-free fabric. Alcohol disinfects the hood in the drying process known as **desiccation.** Do not use a spray bottle, as alcohol can damage the HEPA filter. Always wet the lint-free towel with alcohol to clean the hood. If the alcohol is not dry, then the surface is not clean. The idea behind the lint-free fabric is to reduce the amount of lint particles or other contaminants that can be brought into the clean room. If the specially designed paper towels are not available, you may use gauze. Under no circumstances should you use regular or industrial paper towels; they produce excessive lint.
4. Starting at the IV pole, wipe all surfaces of the pole from left to right with sterile 70% IPA.

(continued)

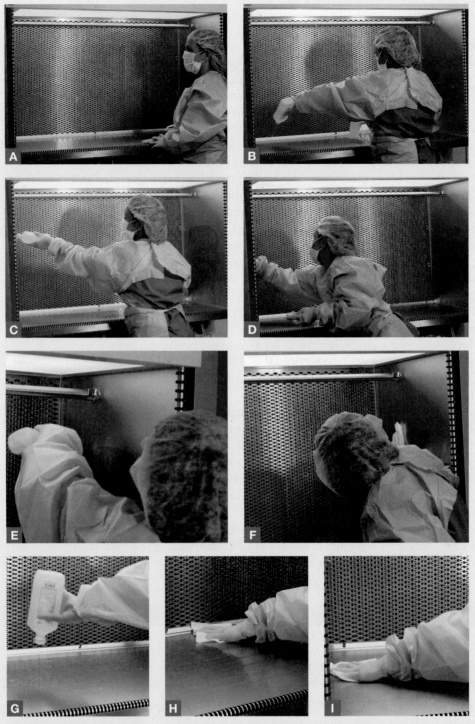

FIGURE 2-6 Cleaning the LAFH

5. After you clean the pole, clean the sides of the hood. Starting at the back of the hood, wipe sides in a vertical fashion (top to bottom) using overlapping strokes. Repeat on the opposite side.

6. To clean the work surface, start in the back corner and clean the surface using horizontal (right to left) overlapping strokes from the back of the work surface to the outer edge.

7. Document the hood cleaning as required by facility.

Cleaning and Disinfecting the Vertical Laminar Flow Hood or BSC

The procedure for cleaning and disinfecting the vertical laminar flow hood or BSC is as follows:

1. Wash the entire hood walls and surface with sterile water to remove salt, starch, sugar, and/or proteins.
2. To clean and disinfect a vertical laminar flow hood or biological safety cabinet, clean from the top down, from the back to the front opening. Using sterile 70% IPA, wet the lint-free towel and begin with the IV pole, cleaning all sides.
3. After you clean the IV pole, clean the back surface of the hood from the top to the bottom with overlapping horizontal strokes. Then clean both sides and the front using the same technique.
4. Last, clean the work surface, from back to front using overlapping horizontal strokes.

Aseptic compounding is best performed with high-quality components and equipment and knowledgeable personnel. Maintaining an aseptic environment is equipment, labor, and management intensive, but it is not technically challenging. The goal of the aseptic environment is to prevent cross-contamination. Since contaminating bacteria are found everywhere, including fingertips, bench tops, and countertops, it is important to minimize contact with these contaminating surfaces.

It is highly important for the pharmacy technician to be aware of and practice proper cleaning procedures as well as aseptic techniques. Cleaning equipment after each use is standard practice regardless of where the compounding is being done.

Other Supplies

Other supplies commonly found in or near a clean room for use include the following:

- Sink with hot and cold running water convenient to the compounding area
- Appropriate disposal or sharps containers for used needles, syringes, and so on, and, if applicable, for infectious wastes and cytotoxic waste from the preparation of chemotherapy agents
- Refrigerator/freezer with a thermometer
- Infusion devices, if appropriate
- Disposable needles, syringes, and other supplies needed for aseptic admixture
- Disinfectant cleaning solutions
- Hand washing agent with germicidal action
- Disposable, lint-free towels or wipes
- Appropriate filters and filtration equipment
- Disposable masks, caps, gowns, and sterile disposable gloves if applicable

The Dressings (Garb)

Clean garments that are relatively particulate free should be worn when working in the sterile preparation area.

Personal Protection Equipment

Personnel who enter the sterile product compounding area are required to wear the appropriate personal protection equipment (PPE) while working under the hood (Figure 2-7).

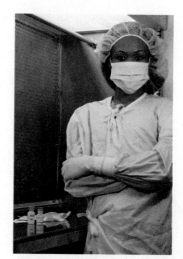

FIGURE 2-7 IV Technician dressed in sterile clothing

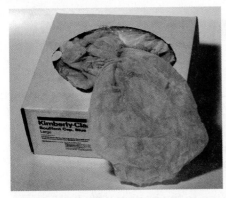

FIGURE 2-8 Hair Cover

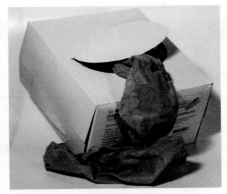

FIGURE 2-9 Shoe Covers

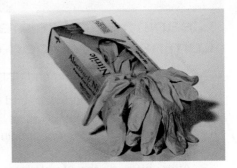

FIGURE 2-10 Gloves

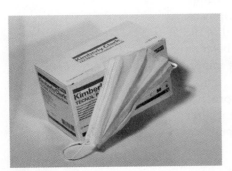

FIGURE 2-11 Masks

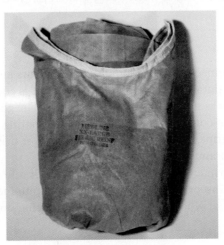

FIGURE 2-12 Gown

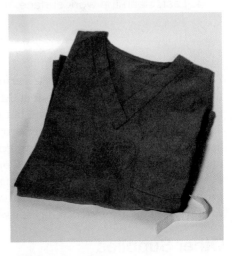

FIGURE 2-13 Scrubs

PPE includes the following:

- **Hair cover**—a surgical cap to cover the hair and prevent the addition of extra particulates in the compounding areas (Figure 2-8).
- **Shoe covers**—to cover the shoes and prevent the addition of extra particulates and any dirt from falling off of the shoes in the clean room (Figure 2-9).
- **Gloves**—to cover the hands and prevent the transfer of contaminants from places such as under the fingernails, as well as to protect any wounds on the hands such as minor scratches (Figure 2-10).
- **Mask**—to cover the mouth and nose and prevent the introduction of saliva and mucus particulates (Figure 2-11).
- **Beard cover**—to be worn by anyone with facial hair (moustache, beard, goatee, unshaven, etc.) to prevent the introduction of hair or skin cell particulates.
- **Gown**—to cover street clothes before entering the clean room to prevent the addition of extra particulates (Figure 2-12).
- **Scrubs**—the preferred clothing in a clean room, designed to be low particulate and can be sterilized by the institution; in a clean 100 room, only scrubs may be worn (Figure 2-13).

Compounding Supplies

There are numerous supplies needed for compounding, and a discussion of each follows.

Alcohol Pads

Alcohol pads are kept close by at all times during preparation and are used constantly for wiping down such things as vial tops (Figure 2-14).

Needles

Needles are used to puncture containers and withdraw or inject fluid. There is a variety of different needle gauges and lengths (Figure 2-15). Needles are disposable and sterile and are not made to be reused or recycled. All parts of the needle must remain sterile.

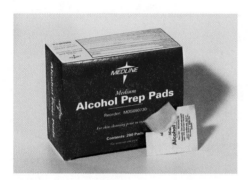

FIGURE 2-14 Alcohol Pads

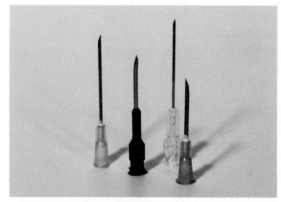

FIGURE 2-15 Needles (various)

Parts of a Needle (Figure 2-16)

- **Lumen**—the hollow space inside a needle
- **Bevel**—the sharp pointed end of the needle
- **Bevel Heel**—the opposite of the bevel; the rounded bottom part of the needle
- **Bevel tip**—the point of the needle
- **Shaft**—the part of the needle between the bevel heel and the hub
- **Hub**—the part of the needle that attaches to the syringe

Needle Length

Different types of injections need different lengths of needles. Sizes may range from ⅜ to 3½ in. or longer (Figure 2-17).

Gauge

Gauge refers to the size of the opening of a needle. The larger the needle's gauge, the smaller is the opening; the smaller the needle's gauge, the larger is the opening. For example, a 25-gauge needle has a very small opening, whereas an 18-gauge needle has a large opening. Needle gauge sizes range from 30 to 16 (Figure 2-18).

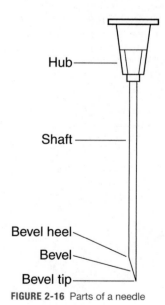

FIGURE 2-16 Parts of a needle

Syringes

Syringes are used to hold and accurately measure liquid medications and diluents. Syringes used for sterile compounding are disposable and sterile and are not made to be reused or recycled.

Parts of a Syringe (Figure 2-19)

- **Tip**—the part of the syringe where the needle is attached to the syringe. This part should never be touched by anything and must remain sterile.

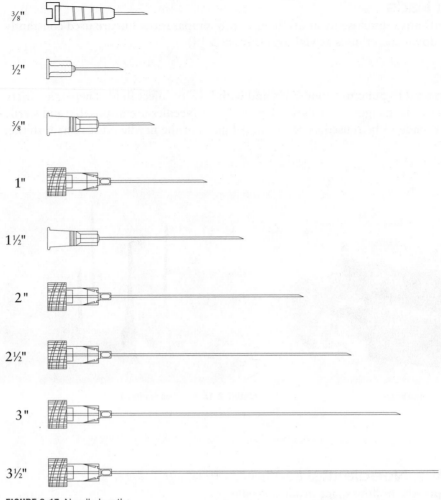

³⁄₈"

½"

⅝"

1"

1½"

2"

2½"

3"

3½"

FIGURE 2-17 Needle lengths

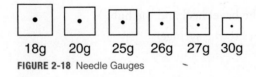

| 18g | 20g | 25g | 26g | 27g | 30g |

FIGURE 2-18 Needle Gauges

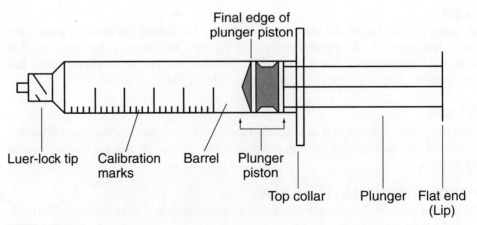

Final edge of
plunger piston

Luer-lock tip   Calibration
marks   Barrel   Plunger
                           piston

Top collar   Plunger   Flat end
                         (Lip)

FIGURE 2-19 Parts of a syringe

- **Barrel**—the part of the syringe where it is usually held. The barrel is where the fluid is held (on the inside). The barrel has the measurement gradations on it.
- **Plunger**—the part of the syringe that slides in and out of the barrel. The plunger should never be touched except on the very end. If the plunger is touched and the plunger goes back into the barrel, the inside of the barrel is now contaminated. The plunger must remain sterile.

Two Types of Syringes

- **Luer lock**—The needle has to be physically screwed onto the syringe (Figure 2-20).
- **Slip tip**—The needle slides onto the end of the syringe (Figure 2-21). Slip tip syringes should never be used to prepare hazardous or chemotherapy medications.

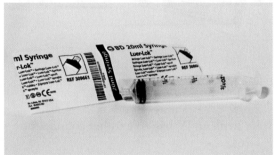

FIGURE 2-20 Luer-lock syringe

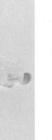

FIGURE 2-21 Slip tip

Miscellaneous

- **Ampule** —This is a sealed container, usually made of glass, containing a sterile medicinal solution, or a powder to be made up in solution, to be used for injection.
- **Single-dose vial (SDV)**—This is a vial that contains no preservatives, and once the container is entered, contaminants may have been introduced and the container is no longer sterile.
- **Sticky mats**—These mats are placed on the floor in the entrance from the anteroom to the clean room. The mats have multiple layers of sticky sheets that can be removed one layer at a time. The mats remove any particulates that may be carried into the clean room on the bottoms of the feet.
- **Vials**—Vials that have preservatives will stay sterile for an extended period of time. The vial's expiration date is determined by the manufacturer's testing. The technician needs to read the package insert on the vial before giving it an expiration date (Figure 2-22).
- **Filters**—Filters are used to remove air, bacteria, fungi, and particulates from a solution. There are three main types:
  - **Membrane filters**—used to remove particulates from a solution. They are attached to the syringe and are used as a form of sterilization (Figure 2-23).

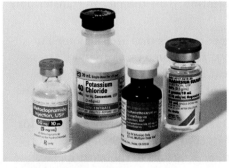

FIGURE 2-22 Vials (various)

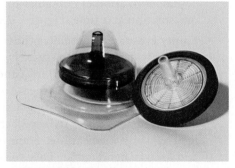

FIGURE 2-23 Membrane filter

- **Depth filters** (filter needles and straws)—used to remove glass shards from a solution. The filter is part of the needle and can be used only once (Figure 2-24 and 2-25).

- **In-line filters**—used as part of the patient's IV set to filter solutions before they enter the patient.

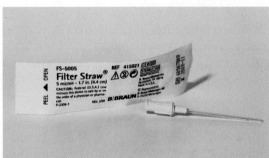
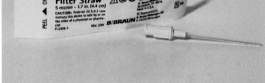

FIGURE 2-24 Filter straw

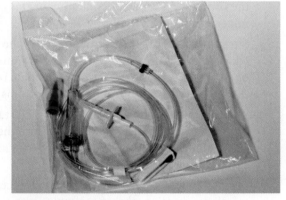

FIGURE 2-25 Filter needle

- **IV tubing**—used to transfer fluid either from an IV bag to another container or from an IV bag to a patient (Figure 2-26).

- **Primary tubing**—used to transfer IV fluid from an IV bag or bottle to a patient. It is usually used by the nursing staff in most facilities; however, if the pharmacy's responsibility is to "prime the tubing," it will use primary tubing. Primary tubing also has many ports so that more than one IV can be administered at the same time (Figure 2-27).

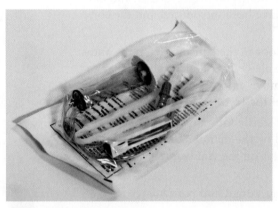

FIGURE 2-26 IV tubing

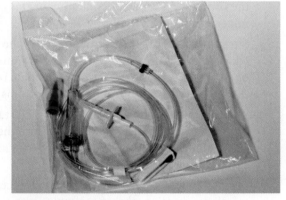

FIGURE 2-27 Primary tubing

- **Vented tubing**—used primarily by pharmacies to transfer the contents of one container to another container for administration. This tubing can transfer only one solution at a time (Figure 2-28).

- **Empty evacuated containers (EECs)**—glass containers that are vacuumed or have a great negative pressure (Figure 2-29). They come in a variety of sizes (150, 250, 500, and 1000 mL) and are great for transferring large volumes from one container to another. Advantages of EECs include the following: There are several different types of glass; they are stronger than plastic; they can be autoclaved; it is easier to inspect the contents; and some are amber colored for light-sensitive medications. Some disadvantages are that they can be very heavy and hard to handle, they have to be vented, and they have rubber stoppers, which can lead to coring.

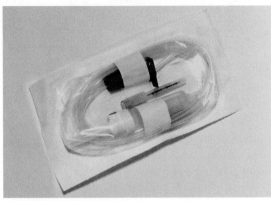

FIGURE 2-28 Vented tubing

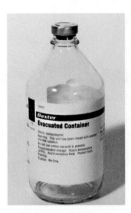

FIGURE 2-29 EEC

- **Viaflex bags**—empty plastic IV bags (Figure 2-30). Viaflex bags have several advantages compared to glass bottles: They are lighter and easier to handle, are less likely to break, and do not require an exchange of air. Some disadvantages are permeability to gases and vapor, leaching of the constituents of the container to the internal contents, transmission of light, masking of chemical incompatibilities, and inability to be thermally sterilized, as they would melt. Viaflex bags are the most common type of IV bag.

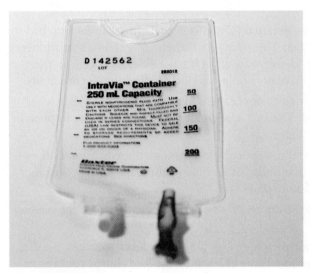

FIGURE 2-30 Viaflex bag

- **Luer-to-Luer connectors**—needle-less system that is very useful when transferring the contents of one syringe to another (Figure 2-31).
- **Dispensing pins**—a needle-less system that allows the contents of a vial to be removed using a Luer-lock syringe. The dispensing pins are also vented, which allows easy transfer of material (Figure 2-32).
- **Minibags or Advantage bags**—an IVPB system allows an entire vial to be aseptically attached to the IVPB without mixing the contents of the vial. These IVPBs can be activated or mixed when the nurse is ready to administer them. The advantage is that they allow for a much longer expiration date.
- **Syringe caps**—used to cover the ends of syringes until they are ready for administration. The pharmacy usually removes the needles so there is less of a chance for needle sticks (Figure 2-33).

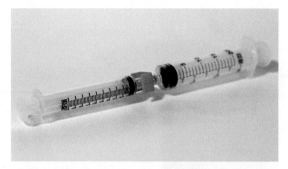

FIGURE 2-31 Luer-to-Luer connector

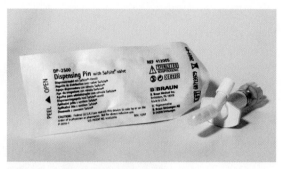

FIGURE 2-32 Dispensing pin

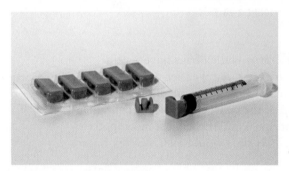

FIGURE 2-33 Syringe cap

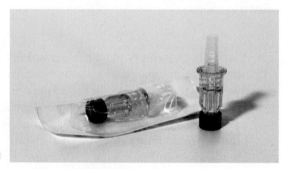

FIGURE 2-34 Port adapter

- **Port adapters (male adapters)**—external IV additive ports that can be attached to the IV additive post of an IV bag. These are great when several different additives are to be added to the IV bag. In this way, all of the needle sticks occur in the port adapter, while the IV additive port only has one needle stick (Figure 2-34).

- **IVA seals (foil port covers)**—used to cover the additive port of an IV bag after the additives have been added. The IVA seal creates a physical barrier to prevent contamination of the IV bag (Figure 2-35).

- **Auxiliary labels**—help to keep the aseptically compounded medication in the correct storage requirements. Examples of auxiliary labels are "protect from light," "refrigerate," and "do not refrigerate."

- **Dark bags**—amber bags placed over an IV, syringe, or bottle to keep the medication out of direct light.

- **Red sharps containers**—containers where any blood products, syringes, needles, glass, or broken glass waste products are thrown away. Red sharps containers require special disposal (Figure 2-36).

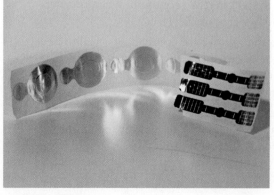

FIGURE 2-35 IVA seal

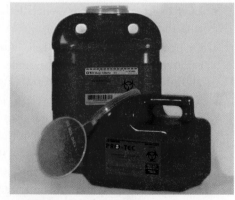

FIGURE 2-36 Sharps container

- **Vented spike adapters**—used to vent glass bottles that are attached to tubing (Figure 2-37).

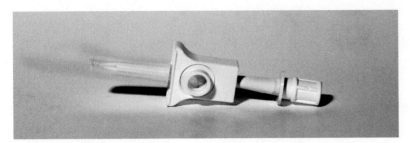

FIGURE 2-37 Vented spike adapter

CONCLUSION

For a technician preparing sterile products, it is important to understand how USP 797 impacts his or her day-to-day activities. USP 797 sets the federal standard for the preparation and compounding of sterile products. USP 797 guidelines provide the preparer with the framework needed to aseptically prepare a sterile product that will not cause harm to the patient.

As with any professional skill, specific equipment and supplies are required to properly prepare sterile products. Thorough knowledge and understanding of each of the standards, guidelines, facilities, equipment, and supplies detailed in this chapter must be acquired in order for someone to become a competent and successful sterile compounding pharmacy technician.

The USP 797 guidelines referenced and explained in this chapter are copyright 2008 United States Pharmacopeial Convention: All rights reserved. Reprinted with permission.

PROFILES OF PRACTICE

One of the topics addressed by USP 797 is personnel training and evaluation. Several states require pharmacy technicians to be certified in sterile product preparation and aseptic technique in order to work in the clean room environment. Requirements vary from state to state, but can include as many as 40 hours of Accreditation Council for Pharmacy Education (ACPE)–accredited continuing education focused on aseptic technique with 20 hours of validated, practical experience.

A number of employers, colleges, and national organizations offer sterile product certification courses for pharmacy technicians, including a national certification course offered by the National Pharmacy Technician Association (NPTA).

CHAPTER TERMS

anteroom the room located right outside the clean room; it is a low-particulate room, which means that it should not contain paper, boxes, or high-particulate matter. Food and drink should not be allowed in this room

desiccation the act of dehydrating or removing water content

germicidal describes an agent that kills pathogenic microorganisms

particulates small matter

single-dose vial (SDV) a vial that contains no preservatives; once the container is entered, contaminants may have been introduced and the container is no longer sterile

vial a small bottle or container that holds products such as injectable medications

CHAPTER REVIEW QUESTIONS

MULTIPLE CHOICE

1. All of the following materials belong in an anteroom except _____.

   a. shoe covers
   b. gowning material
   c. cardboard boxes
   d. sticky mats
   e. antimicrobial soap

2. Which of the following materials do not belong in a compounding area? _____

   a. laminar airflow hood
   b. biological safety cabinet
   c. paper towels
   d. 70% isopropyl alcohol
   e. stainless steel cart

3. An ante area must be at least an _____ environment.

   a. ISO 3
   b. ISO 5
   c. ISO 7
   d. ISO 8

4. What type of syringe is never used to prepare chemotherapy medications?

   a. Luer lock
   b. slip tip

5. The direction of airflow in a biological safety cabinet is _____.

   a. horizontal from back to front
   b. horizontal from front to back
   c. vertical from top to bottom
   d. vertical from bottom to top
   e. horizontal from left to right

6. A filter needle is primarily used for removing _____.

   a. bubbles from a syringe
   b. glass shards and other particulates from a solution
   c. virions and bacteria from a solution
   d. all of the above
   e. a and c only

7. _____ are used for transferring the contents of one syringe to another.

   a. Viaflex bags
   b. Dispensing pins
   c. Luer-to-Luer connectors
   d. Filter needles/filter straws
   e. Metric cylinders

8. _____, which are a needle-less system, are used to remove the contents of a vial into a syringe.

   a. Viaflex bags
   b. Dispensing pins
   c. Luer-to-Luer connectors
   d. Filter needles/filter straws
   e. Luer-lock connectors

9. _____ are empty plastic IV bags that are used as an empty, sterile container.

   a. Viaflex bags
   b. Dispensing pins
   c. Luer-to-Luer connectors
   d. Empty evacuated containers
   e. Vacuums

10. What part of the needle must remain sterile? _____

    a. bevel
    b. shaft
    c. hub
    d. all of the above
    e. only b and c

11. How often should the prefilter be changed? _____

    a. yearly
    b. quarterly
    c. monthly
    d. weekly
    e. biweekly

12. A buffer area must be at least an _____ environment.

    a. ISO 3
    b. ISO 5
    c. ISO 7
    d. ISO 8

13. The PEC must be at an _____ environment.

    a. ISO 3
    b. ISO 5
    c. ISO 7
    d. ISO 8

14. An ISO 5 environment contains no more than _____ particles 0.5 micron or larger per cubic meter of air.

    a. 35.2
    b. 352
    c. 3520
    d. 352,000

15. USP 797 sets standards do not include the _____ of compounded sterile products.

    a. preparation
    b. administration
    c. storage
    d. transportation

LABORATORY ACTIVITIES

1. Practice your understanding of ISO standards for air quality environments.

   a. ISO 3 contains no more than ___32.5___ particles of ___0.5___ or larger per _____ of air.

   b. ISO 4 contains no more than ___352___ particles of ___0.5___ or larger per _____ of air.

   c. ISO 5 contains no more than ___3,520___ particles of ___0.5___ or larger per _____ of air.

   d. ISO 6 contains no more than ___35,200___ particles of ___0.5 micron___ or larger per ___cubic foot___ of air.

   e. ISO 7 contains no more than ___352,000___ particles of ___0.5___ or larger per _____ of air.

   f. ISO 8 contains no more than ___3,520,000___ particles of ___0.5___ or larger per ___cube foot___ of air.

   g. A PEC must have an air environment quality of ISO ___5___.

   h. A buffer area must have an air environment quality of ISO ___7___.

   i. An ante area must have an air environment quality of ISO ___8___.

2. List the three items you will need to clean and disinfect a laminar flow hood.

   a. ___Sterile water___

   b. ___Isopol alcohol 70%___

   c. ___Free towel___

3. Explain the importance of USP 797 to you as a practicing pharmacy technician compounding sterile products.
   ___Is understand and knowledge to become successful and competent___

___for sterile compounding___
_____
_____
_____
_____
_____
_____

4. Gather the supplies needed to disinfect and clean a laminar flow hood. Practice cleaning a horizontal and vertical laminar flow hood. If you do not have a laminar flow hood, practice by explaining the procedures back and forth with your classmate or instructor.
_____
_____
_____
_____

5. Your instructor will display various IV supplies and equipment from the chapter. By sight, name each and explain its use in the IV room.
_____
_____
_____
_____
_____
_____
_____

chapter 3

Aseptic Calculations

LEARNING OBJECTIVES

After completing this chapter, you should be able to:

- Calculate diluent, powder, and final vial volumes for reconstituted powder drugs.
- Calculate IV doses.
- Calculate the volume of electrolytes added to a TPN.
- Calculate IV flow and drip rates.
- Calculate w/w, w/v, and v/v percentage strengths.
- Calculate alligation problems.
- Discuss and calculate dilution technique.

Introduction

For the purposes of this chapter, it is assumed that you have already mastered basic calculations skills. While the use of aseptic technique is necessary when preparing products in the clean room, the calculations that are required are equally important to ensure product integrity and patient safety.

Intravenous Additive Dosage Calculations

Basic sterile compounding involves the transfer of a liquid medication from one container into another container or into an IV solution. To accomplish this, the IV technician must be able to calculate the correct quantity and volume of drug to be withdrawn and transferred using basic ratio and proportion. To determine the dose or volume of the liquid drug to withdraw, set up the ratio proportion as follows:

Drug Concentration Available (What You Have) = Dose or Volume Ordered (What You Need)

example 3.1

Rx: Gentamicin 120 mg IVPB q12h

Drug Available: Gentamicin 40 mg/mL, 2-mL vial

How much drug must be drawn up for each dose?

Set up the ratio proportion: $\dfrac{40 \text{ mg}}{\text{mL}} = \dfrac{120 \text{ mg}}{X \text{ mL}}$

Cross-multiply: $40(X) = 120$

Divide by 40: $X = 3$

Therefore, the technician must withdraw **3 mL** for a 120-mg dose which will require two stock vials.

example 3.2

Rx: Vancomycin 500 mg IVPB q12h

Drug Available: Vancomycin 1 g/10 mL vial

How much drug must be drawn up for each dose?
Convert to like units.

Set up the ratio proportion: $\dfrac{\cancel{1 \text{ g}}\ 1000 \text{ mg}}{10 \text{ mL}} = \dfrac{500 \text{ mg}}{X \text{ mL}}$

Cross-multiply: $1000(X) = 5000$

Divide by 1000: $X = 5$

Therefore, the technician must withdraw **5 mL** for a 500-mg dose. Because the vial contains 1000 mg, the vial contains two doses.

example 3.3

Rx: Cipro 200 mg IVPB BID

Drug Available: Cipro 400 mg/40 mL vial

How much drug must be drawn up for each dose?

Set up the ratio proportion: $\dfrac{400 \text{ mg}}{40 \text{ mL}} = \dfrac{200 \text{ mg}}{X \text{ mL}}$

Cross-multiply: $\qquad$ $400(X) = 8000$

Divide by 400: $\qquad$ $X = 20$

Therefore, the technician must withdraw **20 mL** for a 500-mg dose.

example 3.4

Rx: $\qquad$ Regular insulin 35 units sq now

Drug Available: $\quad$ Regular insulin U-100, 10-mL vial

How much drug must be drawn up in the syringe?

Set up the ratio proportion: U-100 means 100 units/mL. Therefore:

$$\frac{100 \text{ units}}{\text{mL}} = \frac{35 \text{ units}}{X \text{ mL}}$$

Cross-multiply: $\qquad$ $100(X) = 35$

Divide by 35: $\qquad$ $X = 0.35$

Therefore, the technician must withdraw **0.35 mL** for a 35-unit dose.

example 3.5

Rx: $\qquad$ Heparin IV @ 2000 units/hr

Drug Available: $\quad$ Heparin 1000 units/mL, 10-mL vial

$\qquad$ Heparin 5000 units/mL, 1-mL vial

$\qquad$ Heparin 10,000 units/mL, 1-mL vial

The concentration of a standard pharmacy heparin drip is 25,000 units in 1000 mL of 0.9% sodium chloride.

Heparin is a potent anticoagulant and is available in many different concentrations. It is extremely easy to make a mistake when preparing a heparin IV. Therefore, it is critical that technicians be careful and diligent when working with heparin to prevent errors and protect patient safety.

Which size vial(s) would be used, and how much would be withdrawn to prepare a standard heparin drip?

1. If the 1000-units/mL concentration is used:

Set up the ratio proportion: $\qquad \dfrac{1000 \text{ units}}{\text{mL}} = \dfrac{25,000 \text{ units}}{X \text{ mL}}$

Cross-multiply: $\qquad$ $1000(X) = 25,000$

Divide by 1000: $\qquad$ $X = 25$

Therefore, the technician must withdraw **25 mL** for a dose of 25,000 units.

To determine the number of 1000-units/mL 10-mL vials needed:

Set up the ratio proportion: $\qquad \dfrac{10 \text{ mL}}{\text{vial}} = \dfrac{25 \text{ mL}}{X \text{ vials}}$

Cross-multiply: $\qquad$ $10(X) = 25$

Divide by 1000: $\qquad$ $X = 2.5$

Therefore, the technician would pull three vials from stock to prepare the infusion.

2. If the 5000-units/mL concentration is used:

Set up the ratio proportion: $\dfrac{5000 \text{ units}}{\text{mL}} = \dfrac{25,000 \text{ units}}{X \text{ mL}}$

Cross-multiply: $5000(X) = 25,000$

Divide by 5000: $X = 5$

Therefore, the technician must withdraw **5 mL** for a dose of 25,000 units.

To determine the number of 5000 unit/mL 1-mL vials needed:

Set up the ratio proportion: $\dfrac{1 \text{ mL}}{\text{vial}} = \dfrac{5 \text{ mL}}{X \text{ vials}}$

Cross-multiply: $X = 5$

Therefore, the technician would pull five vials from stock to prepare the infusion.

3. If the 10,000-units/mL concentration is used:

Set up the ratio proportion: $\dfrac{10,000 \text{ units}}{\text{mL}} = \dfrac{25,000 \text{ units}}{X \text{ mL}}$

Cross-multiply: $10,000(X) = 25,000$

Divide by 10,000: $X = 2.5$

Therefore, the technician must withdraw **2.5 mL** for a dose of 25,000 units.

To determine the number of 10,000-units/mL 1-mL vials needed:

Set up the ratio proportion: $\dfrac{1 \text{ mL}}{\text{vial}} = \dfrac{2.5 \text{ mL}}{X \text{ vials}}$

Cross-multiply: $X = 2.5$

Therefore, the technician would pull three vials from stock to prepare the infusion.

Which of the foregoing would be the best choice for the IV technician? The choice would depend on the pharmacy's heparin policy. Although each option gives the dose prescribed, option 2 uses the entire contents of each vial without any waste or chance of drawing up too much drug. Another option would be to use two 10,000-units/mL vials (20,000 units) and one 5000-units/mL vials (5000 units). Again, this option would utilize the entire contents of each vial, and there would be no waste. However, some pharmacies discourage the use of multiple strengths of heparin vials or stock only one strength of the drug as a way to decrease the chance of errors.

Diluent, Powder, and Final Volume of Reconstituted Powder Vials

Of course, not all IV drugs are in liquid form. Many drugs, especially antibiotics, are in powder form and must be reconstituted before being administered or added to an IV solution. The volume of diluent needed to reconstitute the drug and the resulting concentration or volume should be written on the vial itself or in the package insert. Most times the pharmacy will have a dilution chart that lists the powder drugs that are stocked along with the diluent volumes and resulting concentrations.

Workplace Wisdom

Powders weighed on an electronic balance are weighed in grams; therefore, milligrams are converted to grams.

When compounding sterile products, the IV technicians often have to change diluent volumes because the dose prescribed cannot be drawn up accurately or safely when the drug is reconstituted according to vial directions. Therefore, IV technicians need to have a complete understanding of the relationship between the diluent volume, powder volume, and final volume or concentration of the vial as presented in the following formula:

$$DV + PV = FV$$

DV = diluent volume
PV = powder volume; the displacement of the powder in the vial, which indicates the volume (if any) that the powder contributes to the final volume
FV = final volume; the total volume of liquid after reconstitution

example 3.6

The 1-g antibiotic vial states "Reconstitute with 3.3 mL of sterile water for a final volume of 4 mL." What is the powder volume in the vial?

Insert the diluent volume of 3.3 mL and the final volume of 4 mL into the formula:

$$3.3 + PV = 4$$

To solve, we need to have the unknown variable (PV) by itself on one side of the equal sign. To do this, we have to subtract 3.3 from each side:

$$3.3 + PV(-3.3) = 4 - 3.3$$
$$PV = 0.7$$

Therefore the powder volume is 0.7 mL.

example 3.7

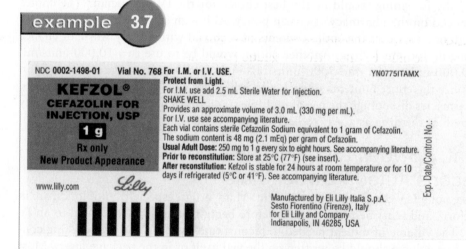

NDC 0002-1498-01   Vial No. 768 For I.M. or I.V. USE.   YN0775ITAMX
Protect from Light.
KEFZOL®   For I.M. use add 2.5 mL Sterile Water for Injection.
CEFAZOLIN FOR   SHAKE WELL
INJECTION, USP   Provides an approximate volume of 3.0 mL (330 mg per mL).
    For I.V. use see accompanying literature.
1 g   Each vial contains sterile Cefazolin Sodium equivalent to 1 gram of Cefazolin.
    The sodium content is 48 mg (2.1 mEq) per gram of Cefazolin.
Rx only   **Usual Adult Dose:** 250 mg to 1 g every six to eight hours. See accompanying literature.
New Product Appearance   **Prior to reconstitution:** Store at 25°C (77°F) (see insert).
    After reconstitution: Kefzol is stable for 24 hours at room temperature or for 10
    days if refrigerated (5°C or 41°F). See accompanying literature.
www.lilly.com   *Lilly*
    Manufactured by Eli Lilly Italia S.p.A.
    Sesto Fiorentino (Firenze), Italy
    for Eli Lilly and Company
    Indianapolis, IN 46285, USA

According to this label, what is the powder volume in the vial?

DV = 2.5 mL
PV = unknown
FV = 3 mL

$$DV + PV = FV$$
$$2.5 + PV = 3$$

$$PV = 3 - 2.5$$
$$PV = 0.5$$

Therefore, the powder volume in the vial is 0.5 mL.

example 3.8

Using the answer in Example 3.7, calculate the diluent volume if you wish to reconstitute the 1-g cefazolin vial to a final volume of 10 mL.

DV = unknown
PV = 0.5 mL
FV = 10 mL

$$DV + PV = FV$$
$$DV + 0.5 \text{ mL} = 10 \text{ mL}$$
$$DV = 10 \text{ mL} - 0.5 \text{ mL}$$
$$DV = 9.5$$

Therefore, to achieve a final volume of 10 mL, the vial should be reconstituted with 9.5 mL of diluent.

example 3.9

If a 500-mg vial is reconstituted with 4.6 mL of diluent for a final concentration of 100 mg/mL, what is the powder volume in the vial?

In this case, the vial's final concentration is given, not the final vial volume. Therefore, the final volume must be calculated using ratio proportion.

Set up the ratio proportion: $\dfrac{100 \text{ mg}}{\text{mL}} = \dfrac{500 \text{ mg}}{X \text{ mL}}$

Cross-multiply: $100(X) = 500$
Divide by 100: $X = 5$

Therefore, the final volume of the 500-mg vial is 5 mL.

Now that we have the final volume, we can calculate the powder volume.

DV = 4.6 mL
PV = Unknown
FV = 5 mL

$$DV + PV = FV$$
$$4.6 \text{ mL} + PV = 5$$
$$PV = 5 \text{ mL} - 4.6 \text{ mL}$$
$$PV = 0.4$$

Therefore the powder volume is 0.4 mL.

Milliequivalents

The milliequivalent (mEq) is a unit of measure commonly used when working with TPNs. While an mEq measurement can look intimidating, it can be treated like any other unit of measure and calculated using ratios and proportions.

example 3.10

ELECTROLYTE	STOCK VIAL	RX ORDER	HOW MANY mL?
NaCl	4 mEq/mL	40 mEq	_____

Using the information provided, set up a ratio and proportion to solve:

$$\frac{4 \text{ mEq}}{1 \text{ mL}} = \frac{40 \text{ mEq}}{x}$$

Cross-multiply: $40 = 4x$

Divide both sides by 4: $X = 10$

So 10 mL of NaCl 4 mEq/mL should be added to the TPN.

Intravenous Flow Rates

IV flow rates are commonly expressed in either milliliters per hour (mL/hr) or drops per minute (gtt/min). When expressed as mL/hr, it is called the IV rate, which is the speed at which an IV solution is infused into a patient. When expressed as gtt/min, it is called the drip rate, which is the speed at which the IV administration set is calibrated to in order to achieve the IV rate. For example, if a patient has an IV ordered at 100 mL/hr, the nurse has to calculate the drip rate so he or she can calibrate the IV administration set to deliver a rate of 100 mL/hr.

Use the following formula to calculate an IV flow rate:

FORMULA

$$\frac{\text{Volume to Be Infused (mL)}}{\text{Infusion Time (hr)}} = \frac{\text{mL}}{\text{hr}}$$

example 3.11

Rx: D5W 1 L q6h. What is the IV rate?

1000 mL/6 hr = 166.67 ≈ 167 mL/hr

IMPORTANT: IV rates should always be rounded to the nearest whole number (mL), as decimal values cannot be accurately measured.

example 3.12

Rx: NS 1 L q8h. What is the IV rate?

1000 mL/8 hr = 125 ml/hr

Rx: LR 500 mL q12h. What is the IV rate?
500 mL/12 hr = 41.667 ≈ 42 mL/hr

Intravenous Frequency or Schedule

An IV frequency or schedule is the time it takes to infuse a specific volume of solution. An IV frequency/schedule is usually expressed in hours. When expressing an IV schedule, do not follow standard rounding rules. Always round the frequency/schedule of an IV down to the nearest whole number in hours, as this will ensure that the patient has enough IV to last over the scheduled period of time.

Use the following formula to calculate an IV frequency or schedule:

FORMULA

$$\frac{\text{Total Volume to Be Infused (mL)}}{\text{IV Rate (mL/hr)}} = \text{q\_hr}$$

example 3.13

Rx: NS 1 L to be infused at 145 mL/hr. What is the frequency of a 1-L IV bag?

$$\frac{1000 \text{ mL}}{145 \text{ mL/hr}} = 6.9\text{hr}$$

Therefore, a 1-L bag will last 6 hr, or the frequency is 6q7h.

example 3.14

What is the frequency of a 500-mL IV bag if the rate of infusion is 50 mL/hr?

$$\frac{500 \text{ mL}}{50 \text{ mL/hr}} = 10\text{hr}$$

Therefore, a 500-mL IV bag will last 10 hr, or the frequency is q10h.

Intravenous Drip Rates

An IV drip rate is used by the caregiver to calibrate the IV administration set to ensure the correct infusion of IV solution. Each IV administration set is labeled with a drop factor (gtt/mL). The drop factor determines how many drops per milliliter are delivered in that particular IV set. Not all IV sets have the same drop factor. Microdrip IV sets are calibrated at 60 gtt/mL, and macrodrip IV sets are calibrated at 10 or 20 gtt/mL. Always ensure you know the proper drop factor before beginning.

Use the following formula to calculate an IV drip rate:

FORMULA

$$\frac{\text{Volume to Be Infused (mL)}}{\text{Infusion Time (min)}} \times \text{IV Set Drop Factor} = \frac{\text{Drops}}{\text{Minute}}$$

example 3.15

Rx: Infuse D5W 500 mL over 4 hr with an IV set with a drop factor of 10 gtt/mL. What is the drip rate?

First, determine the total time to infuse 500 mL:

$$4 \text{ hr} \times 60 \text{ min/hr} = 240 \text{ min}$$

Set up the formula:

$$\frac{500 \text{ mL}}{240 \text{ min}} \times \frac{10 \text{ gtt}}{\text{mL}} = x \frac{\text{gtt}}{\text{min}}$$

Cancel like units before multiplying:

$$\frac{500 \text{ mL}}{240 \text{ min}} \times \frac{10 \text{ gtt}}{\text{mL}} = x \frac{\text{gtt}}{\text{min}}$$

Multiply 500 × 10, then divide by 240, and the resulting answer will be in gtt/min:

$$5000/240 = 20.8 \approx 21 \text{ gtt/min}$$

example 3.16

Rx: Infuse NS 1000 mL over 8 hr. IV set drop factor = 10 gtt/mL. What is the drip rate?

Determine the total time to be infused:

$$8 \text{ hr} \times 60 \text{ min/hr} = 480 \text{ min}$$

Set up the formula:

$$\frac{1000 \text{ mL}}{480 \text{ min}} \times \frac{60 \text{ gtt}}{\text{mL}} = x \frac{\text{gtt}}{\text{min}}$$

Cancel like units before multiplying:

$$\frac{1000 \text{ mL}}{480 \text{ min}} \times \frac{60 \text{ gtt}}{\text{mL}} = x \frac{\text{gtt}}{\text{min}}$$

Multiply 1000 × 60, then divide by 480, and the resulting answer will be in gtt/min:

$$60,000/480 = 125 \text{ gtt/min}$$

example 3.17

Rx: NS 1000 mL, D5W 1000 mL, LR 2000 mL; infuse one bag after the other over 18 hr.

What is the IV rate if the IV set delivers 20 gtt/mL?

First, we need to determine the total volume to be infused:

$$1000 \text{ mL} + 1000 \text{ mL} + 2000 \text{ mL} = 4000 \text{ mL}$$

Now,

$$18 \text{ hr} \times 60 \text{ min/hr} = 1080 \text{ min}$$

Set up the formula:

$$\frac{4000 \text{ mL}}{1080 \text{ min}} \times \frac{20 \text{ gtt}}{\text{mL}} = x \frac{\text{gtt}}{\text{min}}$$

Cancel like units before multiplying:

$$\frac{4000 \text{ \sout{mL}}}{1080 \text{ min}} \times \frac{20 \text{ gtt}}{\text{\sout{mL}}} = x \frac{\text{gtt}}{\text{min}}$$

Multiply 4000 × 20, then divide by 1080, and the resulting answer will be in gtt/min:

$$80{,}000/1080 = 74.07 \approx 74 \text{ gtt/min}$$

Percentage Concentrations

Percentage concentration calculations are used to determine the percentage strength or the amount of active ingredient in a particular preparation. Because percent indicates parts per 100, the percentage strength of a pharmaceutical is an expression of the amount of active ingredient in 100 mL or 100 g of a given final product. When solids are dissolved in liquids, the solid is considered the *solute* and the liquid is considered the *solvent*. When a liquid is mixed with another liquid, the liquid with the smaller quantity is the *solute* and the larger quantity of liquid is the *solvent*. Percentage concentrations of pharmaceuticals may be classified as weight-to-weight (w/w), weight-to-volume (w/v), or volume-to-volume (v/v) percentages as follows:

$\text{w/w\%} = \dfrac{\text{g}}{100 \text{ g}}$ = number of grams of the drug in 100 g of final product, which means that if you have a 10% (w/w) preparation, you have 10 g of active ingredient in every 100 g of final product.

$\text{w/v\%} = \dfrac{\text{g}}{100 \text{ mL}}$ = number of grams of the drug in 100 mL of final product, which means that if you have a 20% (w/v) preparation, you have 20 g of active ingredient in every 100 mL of final product.

$\text{v/v\%} = \dfrac{\text{mL}}{100 \text{ mL}}$ = number of milliliters of the drug in 100 mL of the final product, which means that if you have a 30% (v/v) preparation, you have 30 mL of active ingredient in every 100 mL of final product.

example 3.18

How many grams of dextrose are in 1 L of D50W?

By definition, D50W means that 50 g of dextrose are in 100 mL of final product. Therefore, using the definition of percentage strength, we can set up a ratio proportion to calculate how many grams of dextrose are in 1 L of D50W as follows:

$$\frac{50 \text{ g}}{100 \text{ mL}} = \frac{X \text{ g}}{1000 \text{ mL}}$$

Cross-multiply:

$$100X = 50,000$$

Divide by 100:

$$X = 500$$

Therefore, 1 L of D50W contains 500 g of dextrose.

example 3.19

How many grams of NaCl are in 1 L of normal saline?

If we know that normal saline is 0.9% sodium chloride, by percent definition, there is 0.9 g of sodium chloride in 100 mL of NS. Now, we can calculate the answer by setting up a ratio proportion and solving for X:

$$\frac{0.9 \text{ g}}{100 \text{ mL}} = \frac{X \text{ g}}{1000 \text{ mL}}$$

Cross-multiply:

$$100X = 900$$

Divide by 100:

$$X = 9$$

Therefore, 1 L of NS contains 9 g of sodium chloride.

example 3.20

If there is 0.5 g of active ingredient in 5 g of an ophthalmic ointment, what is the percentage strength (w/w) of the ointment?

For this problem, we calculate the percentage strength and determine how many grams of active ingredient are contained in 100 g of final product if 5 g of final product contain 0.5 g of active ingredient.

Set up the ratio proportion:

$$\frac{X \text{ g}}{100 \text{ g}} = \frac{0.5 \text{ g}}{5 \text{ g}}$$

Cross-multiply:

$$5X = 50$$

Divide by 5:

$$X = 10$$

Therefore, the percentage strength of the ophthalmic ointment is 10%.

example 3.21

If there are 10 mL of active ingredient in NS 500 mL, what is the percentage strength (v/v) of the IV admixture?

Set up the ratio proportion:

$$\frac{X \text{ mL}}{100 \text{ mL}} = \frac{10 \text{ mL}}{500 \text{ mL}}$$

Cross-multiply:

$$500X = 1000$$

Divide by 500:

$$X = 2$$

Therefore, the percentage strength of the IV admixture is 2%.

example 3.22

If 40 g of active ingredient are diluted to 1 L, what is the percentage strength (w/v)?

Set up the ratio proportion:

$$\frac{X \text{ mL}}{100 \text{ mL}} = \frac{40 \text{ g}}{1000 \text{ mL}}$$

Cross-multiply:

$$1000X = 4000$$

Divide by 1000:

$$X = 4$$

Therefore, the percentage strength is 4%.

example 3.23

How much active ingredient is contained in 250 mL of a 12% (v/v) solution?

By definition, 12% (v/v) means that 100 mL of solution contains 12 mL of active ingredient.

Set up the ratio proportion:

$$\frac{12 \text{ mL}}{100 \text{ mL}} = \frac{X \text{ mL}}{250 \text{ mL}}$$

Cross-multiply:

$$100X = 3000$$

Divide by 100:

$$X = 30$$

Therefore, 250 mL of a 12% solution contains 30 mL of active ingredient.

example 3.24

What is the percentage strength (w/v) of a 1 mg/mL epinephrine IV solution?

To determine the percentage strength of a 1 mg/mL solution, we need to find out how much drug is contained in 100 mL.

Set up the ratio proportion:

$$\frac{X \text{ g}}{100 \text{ mL}} = \frac{1 \text{ mg}}{\text{mL}}$$

Cross-multiply:

$$X = 100$$

Therefore, 100 mL contains 100 mg. However, percentage strength is grams per 100 g, not per 100 mg, so we must convert 100 mg to grams.

If 1000 mg = 1 g, then how many grams is 100 mg? We write

$$\frac{1000 \text{ mg}}{1 \text{ g}} = \frac{100 \text{ mg}}{X \text{ g}}$$

Cross-multiply:

$$1000X = 100$$

Divide by 1000:

$$X = 0.1$$

Therefore, the percentage strength of a 1-mg/mL IV solution is 0.1%.

Alligations

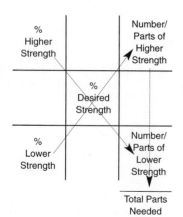

% Higher Strength

% Lower Strength

% Desired Strength

Number/ Parts of Higher Strength

Number/ Parts of Lower Strength

Total Parts Needed

When two different strengths of the same active ingredient are being mixed together, *alligations* are used to calculate the amount of each product needed to produce the desired product. You can easily solve this type of problem by using the alligation grid at left. First, input the amount to be made in the middle square, the higher strength that is available in the top left corner, and the lower strength in the lower left corner. Then take the difference on the diagonals (which should always be a positive number) to determine the number or parts needed. Add the needed parts of the higher strength to the needed parts of the lower strength to determine the total number of parts for the problem. List the parts of each strength over the total parts and multiply each by the total volume desired. For the final answers, read the grid from left to right.

Anytime you are using a solvent or diluent such as water or normal saline (if sodium chloride is not the active ingredient), use a percentage strength of zero.

example 3.25

How much dextrose 70% should be mixed with dextrose 5% to compound 1 L of dextrose 30%?

Set up the alligation grid with the desired concentration in the middle, the higher concentration above, and the lower concentration below, as follows:

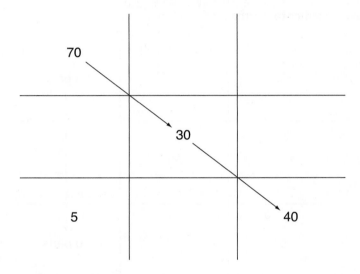

Next, on the diagonal, subtract the desired concentration from the higher concentration and place the result in the lower right corner.

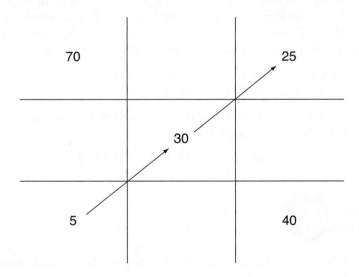

Then, subtract the lower concentration from the desired concentration and place the result in the upper right corner of the grid.

When read from left to right, the grid now shows that you need 25 parts of 70% and 40 parts of 5% dextrose.

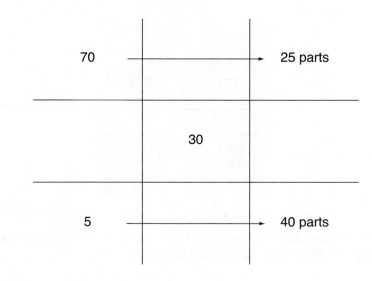

Add the parts together to get the total parts needed:

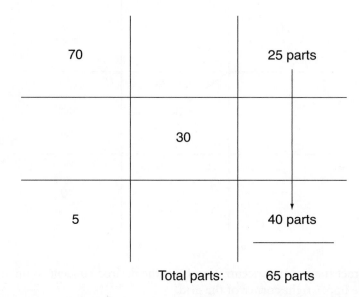

| | Total parts: | 65 parts |

To make this order, you would use 25 parts (out of 65 total parts) of the 70% dextrose and 40 parts (out of 65 total parts) of the 5% dextrose. Since we know the proportion required and the total amount needed, we can calculate an actual amount required of each product by multiplying the total quantity by the proportion needed.

Quantity of 70% needed: 1000 mL × 25/65 = 384.6 mL
Quantity of 5% needed: 1000 mL × 40/65 = 615.4 mL

To check your answer, add both calculated volumes together, which if correct, should add up to the volume desired:

$$384.6 \, \text{mL} + 615.4 \, \text{mL} = 1000 \, \text{mL}$$

example 3.26

How much 91% isopropyl alcohol and sterile water will be needed to prepare 1 gallon of sterile 70% isopropyl alcohol?

Set up the alligation grid with the desired concentration in the middle, the higher concentration above, and the lower concentration below, as follows:

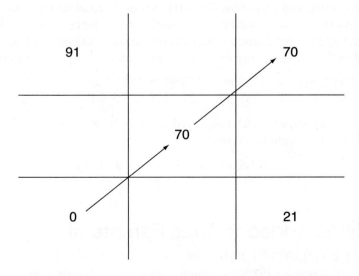

Next, on the diagonal, subtract the desired concentration from the higher concentration and place the result in the lower right corner.

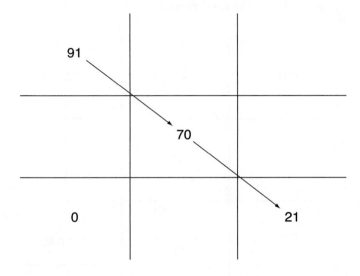

Then, subtract the lower concentration from the desired concentration and place the result in the upper right corner of the grid.

When read from left to right, the grid now shows that you need 70 parts of 91% alcohol and 21 parts of sterile water.

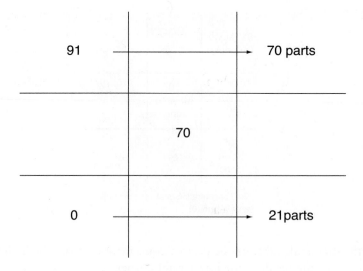

Add the parts together to get the total parts needed:

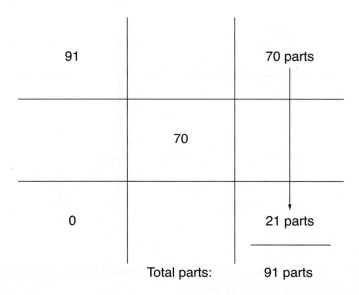

To make this order, you would use 70 parts (out of 91 total parts) of the 91% alcohol and 21 parts (out of 91 total parts) of sterile water. Since we know the proportion required and the total amount needed, we can now calculate an actual amount required of each product by multiplying the total quantity by the proportion needed.

Quantity of 91% needed: 3785 mL × 70/91 = 2911.5 mL
Quantity of 5% needed: 3785 mL × 21/91 = 873.5 mL

To check your answer, add both calculated volumes together, which, if correct, should add up to the volume desired:

$$2911.5\,\text{mL} + 873.5\,\text{mL} = 3785\,\text{mL}$$

Electrolytes Added to Total Parenteral Nutrition Preparations

Total parenteral nutrition (TPN) is administered intravenously when the nutritional needs of a patient cannot be met via oral consumption of nutrients. TPNs are a balanced admixture of carbohydrates, protein, fats, minerals, electrolytes, vitamins, and water.

Electrolytes are charged ions in solution that are important in maintaining acid-base balance in body fluids, controlling body water volume, and regulating metabolism. Milliequivalents are often the unit of measure for electrolyte drug concentrations.

Electrolytes are available in stock vials with the concentration noted on the vial. To determine the volume needed, simply note the total strength of ingredient required and divide by the concentration noted on the vial.

example 3.27

Determine the volume needed for each of the following electrolytes.

NaCl

Stock vial concentration = 4 mEq/mL

Milliequivalents ordered = 60 mEq

Volume needed: 60 mEq/4 mEq = 15 mL

Na phosphate

Stock vial concentration = 4 mEq/mL

Milliequivalents ordered = 40 mEq

Volume needed: 40 mEq/4 mEq = 10 mL

K acetate

Stock vial concentration = 2 mEq/mL

Milliequivalents ordered = 24 mEq

Volume needed: 24 mEq/2 mEq = 12 mL

$MgSO_4$

Stock vial concentration = 4 mEq/mL concentration = 4 mEq/mL

Milliequivalents ordered = 35 mEq

Volume needed: 35 mEq/4 mEq = 8.75 mL

Na acetate

Stock vial concentration = 2 mEq/mL

Milliequivalents ordered = 12 mEq

Volume needed: 12 mEq/2 mEq = 6 mL

KCl

Stock vial concentration = 2 mEq/mL

Milliequivalents ordered = 42 mEq

Volume needed: 42 mEq/2 mEq = 21 mL

K phosphate

Stock vial concentration = 4.4 mEq/mL

Milliequivalents ordered = 13 mEq

Volume needed: 13 mEq/4.4 mEq = 2.95 mL

Ca gluconate

Stock vial concentration = 0.465 mEq/mL

Milliequivalents ordered = 20 mEq

Volume needed: 20 mEq/0.465 mEq = 43.01 mL

TPNs contain a number of electrolytes that start out in a stock vial. The milliliters required are drawn into a syringe and injected into a TPN bag through the injection port and prepared for IV administration. After calculating the volume of each component needed for the order, add them up to determine the total volume of electrolytes. In Example 3.27, the total volume of electrolytes, from Na phosphate to Ca gluconate, is 103.7 mL.

Dilution Technique

A few medications have such a minute dose that dilution is required. The general procedure for diluting is to dilute 1 mL of the concentrate with 9 mL of sterile water for injection. Then take 1 mL of that concentration and further dilute it with 9 mL of sterile water for injection. To further dilute, take 1 mL of that concentration and dilute it with 9 mL of sterile water for injection, and so on. A new empty sterile vial is utilized for each subsequent dilution.

example 3.28

Rx: Insulin dilution to 10 U/mL

Take 1 mL from a stock vial containing 100 U/mL and inject it into an empty sterile vial. Add 9 mL of sterile water for injection. What is the resulting concentration?

Answer: 100 U/10 mL or 10 U/1 mL.

If a patient requires a dose of three units once daily, what volume should be injected?

$$\frac{10\ U}{1\ mL} :: \frac{3\ U}{x\ mL} = 0.3\ mL$$

CONCLUSION

Clearly, many calculations are required when working with sterile products; this chapter has covered the most common calculations a pharmacy technician will encounter in this setting, but it cannot replace a strong comprehension of all pharmacy calculations. Many aseptic calculations seem overwhelming and intimidating at first glance; however, nearly all are solved using simple algebraic principles or ratios/proportions.

CHAPTER REVIEW QUESTIONS

MULTIPLE CHOICE

1. Rx: Penicillin G potassium 250,000 units IVPB q6h. After reconstitution, the vial concentration is 5,000,000 units/20 mL. How many milliliters of penicillin should be drawn up for each IVPB?
   a. 0.5 mL
   b. 1 mL
   c. 4 mL
   d. 20 mL

2. Rx: Dexamethasone 12 mg IVP
   Drug available: Dexamethasone 4 mg/5 mL

How many milliliters would be needed to be drawn up for one dose?
   a. 3 mL
   b. 2.4 mL
   c. 10 mL
   d. 15 mL

Rx: Heparin 40,000 units in D5W 1000 mL.
Drug available: Heparin 10,000 units/mL 2 mL single-dose vial

3. How much heparin would be injected into the D5W 1000-mL bag?

   a. 1 mL
   b. 2 mL
   c. 4 mL
   d. 8 mL

4. How many heparin vials would be pulled from inventory to prepare the heparin infusion?

   a. 1
   b. 2
   c. 3
   d. 4

5. A 1-g antibiotic vial states "Reconstitute with 3.4 mL of sterile water for a final volume of 4 mL." What is the powder volume in the vial?

   a. 3.4 mL
   b. 0.6 mL
   c. 4 mL
   d. 4.6 mL

6. A 10-g antibiotic vial states "Reconstitute with 42 mL of sterile water for a final concentration of 1 g/5 mL." What is the powder volume in the vial?

   a. 5 mL
   b. 10 mL
   c. 8 mL
   d. 4 mL

7. A 10-g antibiotic vial states "Reconstitute with 42 mL of sterile water for a final concentration of 1 g/5 mL." What is the final volume in the vial after reconstitution?

   a. 47 mL
   b. 52 mL
   c. 46 mL
   d. 50 mL

8. A 2-g antibiotic vial states "Reconstitute with 8.6 mL of sterile water for a final volume of 10 mL." What is the concentration of the vial after reconstitution?

   a. 2 g/8.6 mL
   b. 232.6 mg/mL
   c. 0.234 mg/mL
   d. 200 mg/mL

9. How much 4-mEq/mL NaCl must be drawn up for a 27-mEq dose?

   a. 6.7 mL
   b. 6.8 mL
   c. 7.6 mL
   d. 8.6 mL

10. What is the IV flow rate of 1000 mL infused over 12 hr?

    a. 100 mL/hr
    b. 83 mL/hr
    c. 84 mL/hr
    d. 101 mL/hr

11. What is the IV flow rate of 3 L infused over a 24-hr period?

    a. 8 mL/hr
    b. 250 mL/hr
    c. 120 mL/hr
    d. 125 mL/hr

12. How long will a 1-L IV bag last if it is to be infused at a rate of 50 mL/hr?

    a. 20 hr
    b. 6 hr
    c. 10 hr
    d. 8 hr

13. Rx: NS 1 L at 125 mL/hr
    IV set: 10 gtt/mL
    What is the drip rate of this IV?

    a. 125 gtt/min
    b. 20.8 gtt/min
    c. 10 gtt/min
    d. 21 gtt/min

14. What is the drip rate of 3 L of solution infused over 24 hr using an IV set with a drop factor of 60 gtt/mL?

    a. 60 gtt/min
    b. 120 gtt/min
    c. 125 gtt/min
    d. 1440 gtt/min

15. How many grams of sodium chloride are contained in 250 mL of D5 ½NS?

    a. 125 g
    b. 1.125 g
    c. 11.25 g
    d. 1.25 g

16. How many grams of dextrose are contained in 500 mL of D70W?

    a. 70 g
    b. 500 g
    c. 7.14 g
    d. 350 g

17. If you use 4 g of drug to prepare 250 mL of an IV solution, what is the percentage strength of the final product?

    a. 10%
    b. 1.6%

c. 1.1%
d. 4%

For Questions 18–19 use the following information:

Rx: D50W 500 mL

Available: D70W and D10W

18. How much D70W must be used?
    a. 250 mL
    b. 167 mL
    c. 375 mL
    d. 333 mL

19. How much D10W must be used?
    a. 167 mL
    b. 125 mL
    c. 333 mL
    d. 250 mL

For Questions 20–21 use the following information:

Rx: Dextrose 20% 2 L

Available: D70W and SWFI

20. How much D70W must be used?
    a. 0.57 mL
    b. 1.43 mL
    c. 1429 mL
    d. 571 mL

21. How much SWFI must be used?
    a. 0.57 mL
    b. 1.43 mL
    c. 1429 mL
    d. 571 mL

22. Rx: TPN with electrolytes
    How many milliliters of each of the following
    electrolytes should be injected into the TPN bag?
    a. NaCl
       stock vial: 4 mEq/mL
       ordered: 24 mEq
       needed: 6 mL
    b. Na phosphate
       stock vial: 4 mEq/mL
       ordered: 32 mEq
       needed: 8 mL
    c. K acetate
       stock vial: 2 mEq/mL
       ordered: 12 mEq
       needed: 6 mL

LABORATORY ACTIVITIES

All of the following laboratory activities utilize Meducation
training vials, powders, and ampules.

d. Magnesium sulfate
   stock vial: 4 mEq/mL
   ordered: 40 mEq
   needed: 10 mL
e. KCl
   stock vial: 2 mEq/mL
   ordered: 27 mEq
   needed: 13.5 mL
f. K phosphate
   stock vial: 4.4 mEq/mL
   ordered: 25 mEq
   needed: 6 mL
g. Ca gluconate
   stock vial: 0.465 mEq/mL
   ordered: 18 mEq
   needed: 39 mL
h. What is the total volume of electrolytes to be
   added? 83.5 mL

23. Rx: Prostaglandin E 10 mcg/mL
    If the stock container of prostaglandin E is 100
    mg/mL, how many 9-mL dilutions are required to
    prepare the ordered concentration?

24. Rx: Ceftriaxone 500 mg IVPB in D5W 50 mL,
    infuse over 30 min q12h.
    The 2-g ceftriaxone vial states that if you reconsti-
    tute with 8.6 mL, the resulting final volume of the
    vial is 10 mL.

    a. How much diluent would be added to obtain a
       vial concentration of 1 g/10 mL?

    _____

    b. If the vial is diluted to 1 g/10 mL, how much
       drug would be drawn up for one dose?

    c. How many doses are available in one 2-g vial?

    d. How many vials would be needed to prepare a
       7-day supply?

    e. If you were preparing a 7-day supply, how
       many 20-mL vials of sterile water would you
       need to reconstitute the ceftriaxone vials?

    f. If the 500-mg dose is added to D5W 50 mL,
       what is the total volume of one IVPB?

1. Calculate the volume you would withdraw from
   the vial for the prescribed dose and determine
   the size of syringe you would use to prepare
   the dose.

DRUG	PRESCRIBED DOSE	DOSE VOLUME	SYRINGE SIZE: 1, 3, 5, 10, 20, 30, 60
Liquid 25 mg/mL 10 mL	240 mg IV		
Liquid 50 mg/mL 30 mL	225 mg		
Liquid 330 mg/mL 50 mL	4950 mg		
Liquid 50 mcg/mL 2 mL	90 mcg		
Liquid 100 mg/mL 5 mL	390 mg		
Liquid 25 mg/mL 10 mL	60 mg		
Liquid 50 mg/mL 30 mL	1.1 g		
Liquid 330 mg/mL 50 mL	13.53 g		
Liquid 50 mcg/mL 2 mL	25 mcg		
Liquid 100 mg/mL 5 mL	0.46 g		

2. Calculate the volume of insulin to be withdrawn from the vial for the prescribed dose.

INSULIN	PRESCRIBED DOSE (UNITS)	DOSE VOLUME
Regular, 100 U/mL	23	
NPH, 100 U/mL	43	
70/30, 100 U/mL	56	
Lantus, 100 U/mL	65	
Regular, 100 U/mL	18	
NPH, 100 U/mL	53	
70/30, 100 U/mL	37	
Lantus, 100 U/mL	77	

3. Determine which strength of heparin would be used, calculate the dose volume you would withdraw from the vial for the prescribed dose, and determine the size of syringe you would use to prepare the dose.

Available: Heparin 1000 U/mL 10-mL vial and heparin 10,000 U/mL 5-mL vial.

PRESCRIBED DOSE (UNITS)	STRENGTH OF HEPARIN	DOSE VOLUME	SYRINGE SIZE: 1, 3, 5, 10, 20, 30, 60
2,500			
25,000			
10,000			
800			
35,000			
3,500			
2,700			
20,000			

4. Based on the IV order, calculate:

   a. Concentration that you would dilute the vial

   b. Diluent volume

   c. Volume to withdraw to prepare prescribed dose

   d. Number of vials needed to prepare 24-hr supply of IVs

Drug available: 1-g powder vial. Directions read: For IM use, dilute with 2.5 mL for a concentration of 330 mg/mL. For IV use, dilute with 9.5 mL for a concentration of 100 mg/mL or dilute with 4.5 mL for a concentration of 200 mg/mL.

INTRAVENOUS ORDER	CONCENTRATION	DILUENT VOLUME	DOSE VOLUME	NUMBER OF VIALS NEEDED TO PREPARE 24-HR SUPPLY
500 mg IVPB q12h				
750 mg IVPB TID				
1.5 g IM BID				
0.8 g IVPB q6h				
250 mg IVPB q3h				
100 mg IM q8h				
2000 mg IVPB q6h				
500 mg IM q24h				
1200 mg IVPB QID				
250 mg IM q12h				

Properties of Sterile Products

After completing this chapter, you should be able to:

- Explain the cautions associated with microbial contamination.
- Understand the pH range and why it is important.
- Explain the concepts of compatibility and stability.
- Explain the differences among tonicity, osmolarity, and osmolality.

Introduction

Although sterile products may be compounded for use as inhalants, enterals, topicals, ophthalmics, and otics, the primary focus of this book is on IV aseptic preparations and technique. Although sterile IV products are the most common type of sterile preparation that a pharmacy technician will compound, the fundamental knowledge acquired will apply to all types of sterile preparations.

We cannot emphasize enough the importance of preparing a sterile product that is free from particulates, pyrogens, and other contaminants. When administered, injectables bypass one of the body's greatest barriers to contamination—the skin. Because of this increased risk, it is extremely important that the pharmacy technician preparing a sterile product understand the consequences of poor technique and dangers to the patient who receives the medication.

The finished sterile product solutions must be free of contamination and be clear, and all medications must be completely dissolved. While some ingredients might be somewhat darker in color, there should not be anything floating in the final product—for example, rubber from the **coring** of a vial or solid matter caused by a chemical reaction between the ingredients.

Compounders who prepare sterile products must be fully aware of these considerations. We will discuss some of the most important topics in this chapter.

Particulate Matter

Particulate matter is any solid substance floating in an IV solution that should not be there. Particulates can include, rubber, glass, fibers, or undissolved drug. If the needle is not inserted correctly into the vial's stopper, rubber can break off and be transferred into the IV solution. Whenever the rubber stopper breaks off into the vial, it is called coring. Often when an ampule is opened, glass particles will fall to the bottom of the ampule and can be transferred into an IV solution if the preparer does not use a filter needle. Fibers can be transferred into an IV if the preparer opens a syringe, needle, or alcohol swab over an uncapped needle and syringe. The technician can also transfer undissolved drug into an IV if the additive is not allowed to properly dissolve before transfer. Such particulate matter injected into the vein can lodge and block blood flow or cause inflammation and possible infection (sepsis), as foreign matter has invaded the body. The technician needs to be certain to visually inspect every product he or she prepares for "floaties" or other unusual differences that should not be present, regardless of how many times he or she makes a product.

Workplace Wisdom

Do not take anything for granted or become comfortable enough to not perform a visual check. The pharmacist signing off on the final product will expect you have done this and will be looking for the same as an additional safety precaution and as part of the multiple-check procedure.

PH, Acids, and Bases

The term pH refers to a measure of the acidity or alkalinity of a solution. The *p* stands for *potenz*, meaning "potential to be," and the *H* is for *hydrogen*. The pH scale ranges from 0 (extremely acidic) to 14 (extremely alkaline), with 7.0 being neutral. A neutral solution is neither too **acidic** nor too **alkaline** (basic). With few exceptions, life exists in a fairly narrow range of pH. Therefore, pH is considerably important in understanding normal cellular functions and values, as well as the relationship between acids and bases.

Bases are substances that increase the number of hydroxide ions (OH^-) and thus remove hydrogen ions. By reducing the concentration of hydrogen atoms, bases raise the pH. Thus, as the H^+ concentration increases, the pH decreases. The more H^+ in solution, the more acidic the solution becomes and the lower the pH falls. As the H^+ concentration increases, the pH decreases, thus becoming more acidic (Figure 4-1).

The pH Scale

The pH scale is logarithmic; a decrease of 1 unit on this scale represents multiplying acidity 10 times. For example, bleach is 10 times as basic as soapy water. Acid rain is 100 times as acidic as urine. A solution with a pH of 6.9 or below is considered an acid; anything with a pH of 7.1 and above is considered an alkali or a base.

The pH of a solution is important because it could affect how products react together. When a product reacts, it can cause precipitation, heat, gas, or cloudiness. Because medications are considered chemicals, mixing certain drugs together can change the pH of a solution, sometimes making them incompatible. When a solution becomes incompatible, precipitation or crystallization can occur.

Human blood has a pH of 7.4 (slightly alkaline), while most parenteral solutions are slightly acidic, in the pH range of 3.5–6.2. Dextrose 5% water is slightly more acidic than human blood and therefore can sometimes sting a little while being infused.

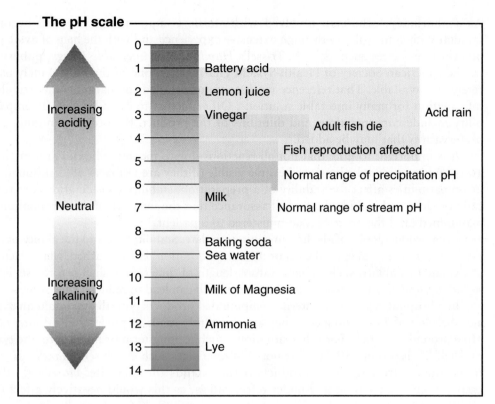

FIGURE 4-1 pH scale

Think of it like this: Ordinary bar soap has a slightly lower pH than that of the human eye. So when it gets in your eyes, it stings! Chemical reactions in the body are very sensitive to even slight changes in the acidity or alkalinity of the body fluids in which they occur. Any departure from the narrow limits of normal H^+ and OH^- concentrations greatly disrupts body functions.

Workplace Wisdom

Think of pH like this: Water can be hot or cold; these extremes of temperature can be neutralized by mixing hot and cold water to even out the temperature. The same theory applies with acids and bases. You can add one or the other to adjust the pH balance.

Compatibility and Stability

Like pH, compatibility is an extremely important factor in preparations. As mentioned, sometimes incompatibility can result in precipitation or crystallization, but sometimes incompatibility is not always visible. Many drugs when mixed together can interact with each other, enhance one another, or even cancel each other out.

Basically, there are three major types of incompatibilities: physical, chemical, and therapeutic.

- **Physical**—This is the easiest incompatibility to identify, as it results in a physical change to the product such as precipitation, cloudiness, presence of heat or cold while mixing, change in color, or separation. It is usually caused by a chemical reaction or improper or incomplete mixing of ingredients.

- **Chemical**—Chemical incompatibility occurs when a chemical reaction causes a change in the molecular structure or activity of the ingredients.

- **Therapeutic**—Therapeutic incompatibility occurs when giving two or more drugs within a short period of time results in decreased effectiveness of one or more of the ingredients.

As a pharmacy technician involved with sterile compounding, you will become familiar with compatibility through extensive experience and with the help of available literature resources such as L. A. Trissel's *Handbook of Injectable Drugs*, published by the American Society of Health-System Pharmacists, one of the most widely used references available. That reference work contains detailed compatibility and stability information for many injectable solutions. Other factors to consider with incompatibility include concentrations and dilutions of the product, the order of mixing, and preservatives that may be added.

It is important to note that not all reactions due to incompatibilities appear right away and can even take hours to become visible (if they are visible at all). Although all incompatibilities affect the stability of a preparation, stability considerations are typically broader and include the overall assurance that the integrity of the formulation is maintained until the product is administered to a patient.

Each product, once made, has an expiration date. Stability refers to the ability of the product to remain stable until used or until the expiration date is reached. Many factors contribute to stability, such as temperature, length of time on the shelf before use, light sensitivity, and chemical reactions over time, which can lead to reduced effectiveness.

In a hospital-type setting, sterile compounded products typically maintain an average shelf life of 24–48 hours, as they are constantly made at predetermined intervals, often around the clock. For other situations, such as long-term or home care, the typical shelf life is around 30 days. As noted in references such as Trissel's *Handbook*, refrigerating or freezing some products often extends the shelf life. However, other preparations cannot be stored under refrigeration, as this would negatively affect the stability and/or compatibility. The key is to understand that each product requires a certain set of instructions regarding preparation and storage. As a professional pharmacy technician, you must be able to research and understand these requirements.

Tonicity

Tonicity refers to the response of cells or tissues to the solutions in which they are immersed. Picture a membrane separating two solutions, one side with a higher solute concentration than the other:

- The side with the higher solute concentration is hypertonic.
- The side with the lower solute concentration is hypotonic.
- If both sides have the same solute concentration, they are isotonic.

The tonicity of an IV fluid dictates whether the solution should be administered by the peripheral or central venous route. Hypotonic and hypertonic solutions may be infused in small volumes and into large vessels, where dilution and distribution are rapid. If a solution's tonicity varies greatly from the normal range, it may cause tissue irritation, pain on injection, or electrolyte shifts.

If cells are placed in a hypertonic solution, movement of water will be out of the cell, causing the cell to shrivel. If cells are placed in a hypotonic solution, movement of water will be into the cell, causing the cell to swell or burst. Tonicity is useful only in reference to a particular cell or tissue.

Isotonic solutions in the human body fall into the range of 280–310 mOsm/L (mOsm is the abbreviation for milliosmoles). Patient safety and comfort are best achieved by utilizing a solution that approximates this isotonic condition.

Osmolality and Osmolarity

Tonicity differs from osmolarity, as osmolarity is an absolute measure of the number of osmotically active solutes in a solution, whereas tonicity is a relative measure based on the osmotic compatibility of a solution with a given cell type.

We begin with some useful definitions. A *mole* (abbreviated *mol* when given with a numerical value) is the amount of a substance that contains 6.022×10^{23} molecules (Avogadro's number). The mass, in grams, of 1 mol of a substance is the same as the number of atomic mass units in one molecule of that substance (that is, the molecular weight of the substance expressed as grams). The mole is the base unit in the International System of Units (SI System) for the amount of a substance. An *osmole* is the amount of a solute that yields, in ideal solution, the number of particles (Avogadro's number) that would depress the freezing point of the solvent by 1.86 K.

Molality of a solution is the number of moles of a solute per *kilogram of solvent.*
Molarity of a solution is the number of moles of solute per *liter of solution.*
Osmolality of a solution is the number of osmoles of solute per *kilogram* of solvent.
Osmolarity of a solution is the number of osmoles of solute per *liter* of solution.

Osmolality depends on the number of particles (active ions or molecules) in a solution. It is commonly expressed as the number of milliosmoles of solute per kilogram of solvent (mOsm/kg).

Osmolarity is a measure of the osmotic pressure exerted by a solution across a perfect semipermeable membrane (one that allows free passage of water and completely prevents movement of solute) compared to pure water. It is commonly expressed as the number of milliosmoles of solute per liter of solution (mOsm/L).

CONCLUSION

Sterile products have special, unique properties that must be taken into consideration. Among the most crucial properties are pH, compatibility, stability, tonicity, osmolarity, and osmolality. Additional information on these properties is available in a number of pharmacy reference books, which should be available at any pharmacy preparing sterile products.

CHAPTER TERMS

acidic describes a substance that increases the concentration of hydrogen ions (lowers the pH); an acidic substance is called an acid

alkaline describes a substance that decreases the concentration of hydrogen ions (raises the pH); an alkaline substance is called a base

coring transferring part of the rubber stopper of a vial or container into a solution bag because of improper needle stick

isotonic describes a solution in which body cells can be bathed without net flow of water across the semipermeable cell membrane; also describes a solution with the same tonicity as another solution.

osmolality the concentration of solute in a solution per unit of solvent; commonly expressed as milliosmoles per kilogram

osmolarity the concentration of solute in a solution per unit of solution; commonly expressed as milliosmoles per liter

CHAPTER REVIEW QUESTIONS

MULTIPLE CHOICE

1. Water moves out of a cell, causing the cell to shrivel, when the cell is placed in a (an) _____ solution.

   a. isotonic
   b. hypotonic
   c. iso-osmotic
   d. hypertonic
   e. osmolality

2. Water moves into a cell, causing swelling, when the cell is placed in a (an) _____ solution.

   a. hypertonic
   b. isotonic
   c. tonicity
   d. hypotonic
   e. osmosis

3. If particulate matter enters and lodges in a vein, what could be the result? _____.

   a. stroke
   b. inflammation
   c. sepsis
   d. both b and c
   e. both a and b

4. Human blood has a pH of _____.

   a. 10.4
   b. 7.4
   c. 6.4
   d. 4.4
   e. 9.4

5. What are the three major types of incompatibilities? _____.

   a. physical, chemical, therapeutic
   b. therapeutic, psychological, mechanical
   c. chemical, electrical, neurologic
   d. physical, chemical, reactive
   e. therapeutic, medical, physical

6. A neutral solution is _____.

   a. alkaline
   b. acidic
   c. chemically altered
   d. both a and b
   e. none of the above

7. What is the most likely reason that bar soap stings when it gets into the eyes? _____.

   a. Water is added to the soap for lather.
   b. The pH balance is not equal between the eyes and the soap.

   c. The volume of the soap is greater than 5 g.
   d. The osmolarity is under 7.4.
   e. The pH of the soap is at 7.0.

8. In a hospital-type setting, sterile compounded products maintain an average shelf life of _____.

   a. 10–12 hr
   b. 8–12 hr
   c. 4–6 hr
   d. 12–24 hr
   e. 24–48 hr

9. Sterile water has a value of _____ mOsm/L.

   a. 15
   b. 0
   c. 5
   d. 10
   e. −0.5

10. If two solutions have the same solute concentration, they are known as _____.

   a. isotonic
   b. hypertonic
   c. hypotonic
   d. iso-osmotic
   e. permeable

LABORATORY ACTIVITIES

1. Fill in the following chart using IV solutions provided by your instructor or research the Internet.

INTRAVENOUS SOLUTION	pH LEVEL 0—14 (ACIDIC OR ALKALINE)	TONICITY (ISOTONIC, HYPERTONIC, HYPOTONIC)	OSMOLARITY (mOsm/mL)
D5W			
NS			
LR			
D5NS			
D5 ½NS			
D5 ¼NS			
D5LR			

2. Use appropriate reference sources to determine whether the following medications and/or IV solutions are compatible or incompatible if mixed together in an IV preparation. If the medications/solutions are compatible, indicate how long the compatibility lasts. If the medications/solutions are incompatible, indicate what happens if the substances are mixed together.

a. Heparin and dobutamine HCl

_____

_____

b. Bleomycin and D5W

_____

_____

c. Hydroxyzine HCl and aminophylline

_____

_____

_____

d. Meperidine HCl and promethazine HCl

_____

_____

_____

e. Nitroglycerin and potassium chloride

_____

_____

_____

f. Vancomycin and D5W

_____

_____

g. Ampicillin and D5W

_____

_____

h. Calcium gluconate and potassium phosphate

_____

_____

i. Amphotericin B and sodium chloride 0.9%

_____

_____

j. Tobramycin and furosemide

_____

_____

Aseptic Technique

After completing this chapter, you should be able to:

- Explain the importance of and demonstrate proper dressing and hand washing procedures.
- Describe how to properly swab objects with alcohol and use syringes, needles, and vials.
- Demonstrate how to reconstitute a powder in a vial.
- Explain the methods for removing air bubbles from syringes, using transfer needles, and using ampules.
- Demonstrate how to remove fluid from an ampule.
- Discuss the proper steps for preparing a sterile dosage form.

Introduction

Aseptic technique involves manipulating medications, fluids, and solutions and transferring them from one container to another, following stringent guidelines. Its primary goal is to keep cultures, sterile instruments, media, and people free of microbial contamination. Aseptic technique involves many factors such as proper dress, hand washing, and manipulation. This chapter will touch on all of the things a pharmacy technician should know before beginning to work in a clean room and environment.

Being physically able and technically correct to compound a sterile product is only a small part of the skill necessary to be competent in the IV room, however. The IV technician must have a wide variety of knowledge in such areas as terminology and IV room materials and supplies, as well as proficiency with mathematical calculations, quality assurance, routes of administration, and drugs.

Preparation

Appropriate dress (garb) must be worn by all personnel at all times while in the compounding area.

Dressing

USP 797 requires that the personnel performing sterile compounding wear the appropriate personal protective equipment (PPE), and personnel cannot wear jewelry, fingernail polish or artificial nails, or makeup of any kind. All PPE should be made of disposable, nonshedding, low-permeability material. The technician should don PPE (Figure 5-1) and perform actions in the anteroom in the following order:

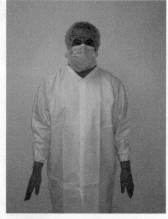

FIGURE 5-1 Proper dressing

1. Put on shoe covers
2. Put on head and facial hair covers
3. Put on face/eye masks
4. Put on eye shields (optional unless preparing hazardous drugs)
5. Aseptically wash hands (see hand washing)
6. Put on nonshedding gown with snug-fitting cuffs
7. Clean hands with waterless, alcohol-based hand scrub
8. Put on sterile, powder-free gloves

All PPE must be removed before leaving the sterile compounding areas. Any PPE that leaves the sterile compounding area is considered contaminated and cannot be reused. Removal of PPE is done in the opposite order from the gowning process. The gown may be reused for the technician's work shift if it has not been contaminated. Head, face, and shoe covers may not be reused and must be replaced.

Hand Washing

Proper hand washing is important because all surfaces of our bodies have bacteria on them. These bacteria, called normal bacterial flora, typically do not affect healthy individuals. However, if the normal bacteria are accidentally given a little food (dextrose) and administered intravenously, they can and will cause an infection. If the patient is ill or **immunocompromised**, these normal bacteria will cause significant harm to the patient. When preparing sterile products, gloves must be worn, and the gloves must also be cleaned and disinfected. Isopropyl alcohol (IPA) 70% or a waterless, alcohol-based hand scrub is used to disinfect hands between hand washings.

Here are some key points for hand washing (Figure 5-2):

- Wash your hands before entering the direct compounding area and donning sterile gloves. Be sure to disinfect gloves by spraying with IPA 70% if the gloves become contaminated.

- Run your hands under warm water and use a nail cleaner and soap to remove all debris from under the fingernails. Nail brushes are not recommended.

- After cleaning under the fingernails, wash hands and forearms for at least 30 sec with soap. USP 797 allows either antimicrobial or nonantimicrobial soap, but the soap should not contain lotion or fragrance. Be sure to wash around and between all fingers and underneath fingernails. Scrub up to the elbow area of each arm, covering the entire area with soap, and rinse completely. Keep fingers pointed upward at all times during hand washing, and allow all water to run down off the elbows.

- Use lint-free paper towels or an electric hand dryer to dry your hands after a hand washing.

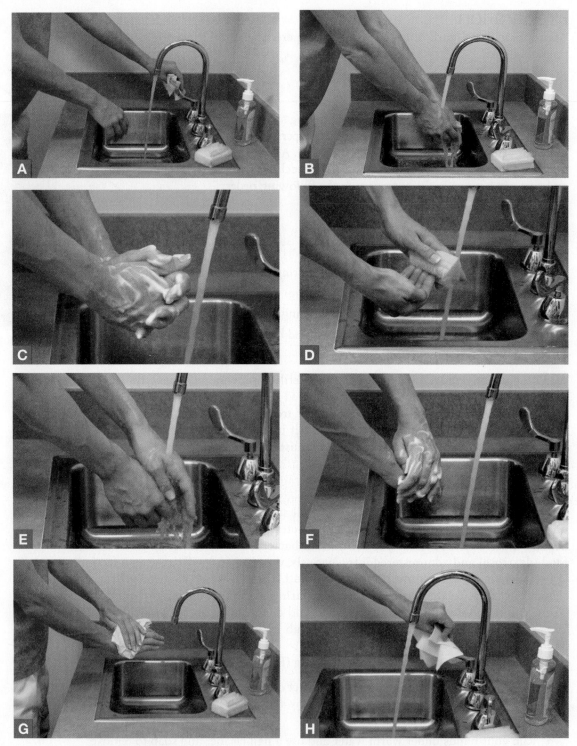

FIGURE 5-2 Proper hand washing

Proper Aseptic Technique

Following is the how-to of aseptic technique and some special considerations for dealing with different products. Read this section carefully, as it is very important for you to become proficient in this task. Refer to this section as often as necessary throughout your pharmacy career. With time and experience, you should become proficient and knowledgeable as you work with many types of fluids, medications, and equipment.

Manipulation

To maintain sterility, you must avoid touching several areas during sterile product manipulations and preparation. Avoid direct contact with any previously swabbed area (vial top, bag port, neck of an ampule), uncapped needles, the hub of the needle, the syringe tip, the syringe plunger, the open tip of a filter or dispensing pin, and the uncapped tip of any tubing.

Basically, any area that may come in contact with the sterile solution should not come in contact with any nonsterile area, including hands, fingers, or any parts that can come in contact with hands and fingers. As a general rule, if the manufacturer has made a cover for a part on a syringe or tubing, that part should remain untouched and sterile. All syringes must have a capped needle or a syringe cap on before you lay them on the hood's surface. Never place uncapped needles or uncovered syringes in the hood.

When withdrawing solution using a dispensing pin, place the dispensing pin cap on a clean alcohol swab. Immediately recap the solution after use and discard the swab.

Swabbing with Alcohol

To guarantee sterility of a critical site that will be punctured/penetrated by a needle, tubing, and so on, you must swab it with 70% isopropyl alcohol. Areas that must be swabbed include the following:

- Vial tops
- Ampule necks
- Tops of bottles
- Ports of any IV or IVPB bags

To properly use an alcohol pad, place the alcohol pad on the area to be swabbed, allowing it to remain for several seconds or until the surface becomes saturated with alcohol. Then make one gentle stroke across the area to be cleaned, moving the swab toward either the side or the front of the hood (not toward the HEPA filter). Use a clean, saturated, unused portion of the swab with each pass. Be certain to allow the alcohol to dry fully before use. Swabbing is effective in two important ways—it removes any physical contaminants such as dust, and it acts as a disinfectant because the evaporation of alcohol, called desiccation, creates sterility.

Using Syringes

Syringes are available in numerous sizes, with volumes ranging from 0.5 to 60 mL. To maximize accuracy, use the smallest syringe size that can hold the desired amount of solution. According to American Society of Health-System Pharmacists guidelines, the total volume being measured must be at least 20% of the total size of the syringe, which is known as the 20% rule. To maintain sterility, two parts of the syringe cannot be touched—the tip and the plunger.

Syringes are single-dose items that you must dispose of in the designated sharps container after use. You must open the syringe package within the clean air space in the PEC in order to maintain sterility. Do not place the syringe's outer packaging on the working surface of the PEC because it will contaminate the DCA. Place the outer covering directly into the garbage after removing the syringe.

Syringes are packaged with either a needle and cap or a protective cover over the tip. Do not remove the protective tip cover until a new needle is ready to be attached on the tip of the syringe. If the syringe does not come with either a protective cap or a capped needle, you must attach a new needle on the syringe immediately, before laying the syringe on the hood's surface.

Many syringes have locking mechanisms, such as a Luer lock at the tip that secures the needle by allowing it to be screwed down onto a threaded ring. When you attach a needle to a Luer-lock-type syringe, you must turn the needle slightly to ensure a tight fit. In other cases, the needle is held on only by friction; these are known as slip tips.

Using Needles

Many needles are available in different sizes and lengths. The width of a needle is measured in gauges. The larger the gauge of a needle, the smaller is the bore (width). For example, a 27-gauge needle has a smaller bore than a 13-gauge needle. Handle a needle only by the protective cover. Avoid touching the hub of a needle. The standard-size needles used in a pharmacy for compounding sterile products vary from 18 to 21 gauge.

Using Vials

Date all vials before you bring them into the hood. Single-dose vials contain no preservatives and should be discarded at the end of the shift. There are several situations in which you must use a preservative-free vial, such as pediatric dilutions, epidurals, and intrathecals. Medications with preservatives can seriously harm patients if administered in these situations.

Multiple-dose vials contain preservatives that allow their contents to be used after the vial has been punctured. These vials each have specific instructions outlined in the package inserts that describe how the vial should be kept (e.g., refrigerated) and for how long the vial remains stable. When an MDV is opened, the date and time opened and the initials of the person opening the vial must be documented on the label of the vial. USP suggests that the MDV beyond-use date is 28 days after opening unless otherwise noted by the manufacturer. However, if you are in doubt, "toss it out," as it is always better to be cautious.

When a vial is pierced by a needle, *cores* or fragments of the rubber stopper can form. To prevent this problem, insert the needle into the rubber stopper with the bevel tip up, then apply a slight lateral pressure (away from the bevel) and downward pressure to insert the needle. Make sure to maintain aseptic technique and avoid shadowing at all times.

Vials are closed-system containers because air cannot flow freely into or out of the vial. Therefore, adding air or fluid to a closed system will cause the vial to become pressurized, also known as *positive pressure*. Positive pressure can cause some spraying of the fluid from the vial or can cause the vial to become leaky. On the other hand, removing air or fluid from the vial can create a vacuum in the vial. If too much of a vacuum is created, it is nearly impossible to remove the contents of the vial aseptically. Therefore, the volume of the fluid to be removed from a vial should be replaced with a slightly smaller volume of air to minimize the vacuum. It is better to have a slight vacuum in a vial because it results in a cleaner withdrawal. Do not add air to gas-producing drugs such as ceftazidime or any chemotherapy drugs.

If the drug within the vial is in a powdered form, it must first be **reconstituted**. Reconstitution is the adding of a diluent to a vial to create a liquid form of the drug. The desired volume of the diluting solution or diluent, usually sterile water for injection (SWFI), is injected into the vial. As the diluent is added, an equal volume of air must be removed to prevent positive pressure from building up within the vial. This is accomplished by allowing an equal amount of air to flow back into the syringe that was used to reconstitute the vial or by using a vented needle. A vented needle allows free flow of air out of the vial during reconstitution, resulting in the release of the built-up positive pressure.

Although most drugs dissolve rapidly when swirled, the IV technician must make sure that a drug is completely dissolved before proceeding. Visually inspect all reconstituted drugs to ensure that the powder is completely dissolved and that there are no cores or other particulate matter in the solution. Carefully inspect the container fully, including as close to the needle entrance as possible and behind any ridges. If you observe or suspect any particulate matter, filter the solution before adding it to the final parenteral product.

Withdrawing from a Vial

This type of manipulation is the simplest and most common. It can be used in almost all manipulations in one form or another.

You must perform a straight draw procedure in the PEC space using proper aseptic technique (Figure 5-3):

1. Follow the proper procedures for dressing and hand washing. Gather all materials needed for the manipulation.
2. Swab the rubber top with alcohol. Allow the alcohol to dry.
3. Make sure the needle is firmly attached to the syringe.
4. Pull the plunger back on the syringe to slightly less than the amount needed to be drawn up.
5. Remove the needle cap. Find the center of the stopper and position the needle with the bevel end up.
6. Holding the needle at an approximate 45-deg angle, insert the needle through the stopper.

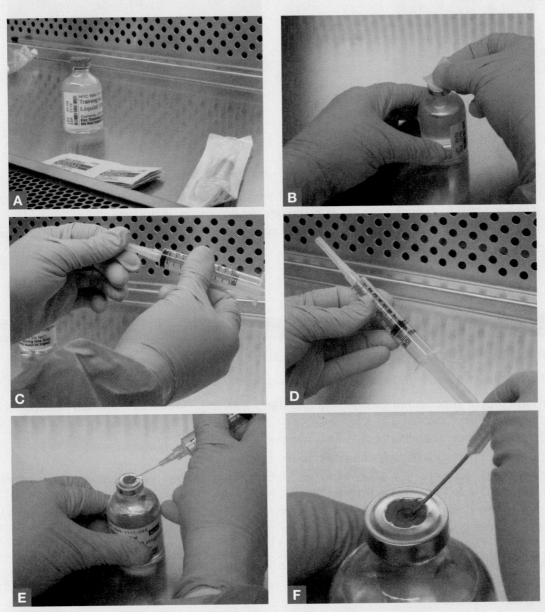

FIGURE 5-3 Straight draw

(continued)

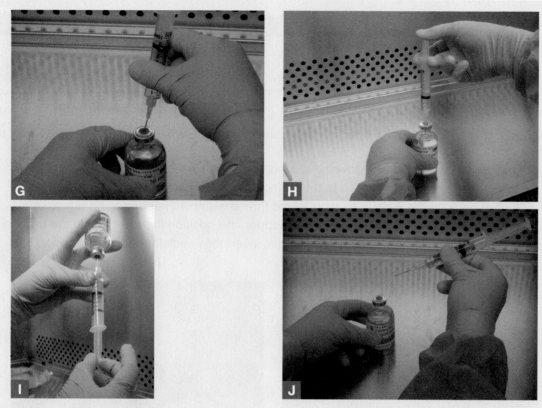

FIGURE 5-3 Straight draw (continued)

7. Gently push the air from the syringe into the vial.
8. Invert the vial and release the plunger. The air in the vial will push the plunger out of the syringe on its own. If needed, pull back on the plunger until the desired amount is withdrawn.
9. Remove any air bubbles by gently tapping on the syringe to force the air to the top of the syringe.
10. Withdraw the needle and carefully recap.

PROCEDURE **5-2**

Reconstituting a Powdered Vial

You must reconstitute a powdered vial in the PEC using proper aseptic technique (Figure 5-4).

1. Follow the proper procedures for dressing and hand washing. Gather all materials needed for the manipulation.
2. Swab all rubber tops with alcohol. Allow the alcohol to dry.
3. Make sure that the needle is firmly attached to the syringe.
4. Draw up the correct amount of diluent needed for the reconstitution using the procedure described earlier with regard to withdrawing from a vial.
5. Pull back on the plunger to clear the neck of the syringe. Remove the needle and replace with a vented needle.
6. Carefully add diluent to the powdered vial.
7. Gently shake or swirl to dissolve. The powder must dissolve completely.
8. Change the vented needle back to a regular needle and carefully remove the desired amount from the vial.
9. Remove any air bubbles.
10. Withdraw the needle and carefully recap.

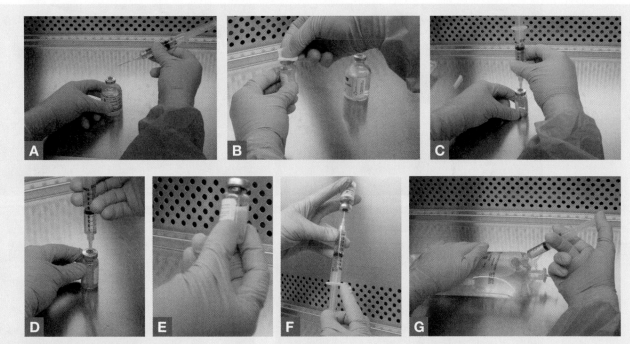

FIGURE 5-4 Reconstitution of a vial

More on Manipulation

Removing Air Bubbles

Often air bubbles will be present in the syringe after you have drawn up the medication (Figure 5-5). To remove air bubbles, draw back on the plunger to allow more air in the syringe. Then carefully rotate the large air bubble around the syringe. The larger air bubble should pick up most of the smaller air bubbles. If air bubbles are left, carefully tap the syringe to dislodge the smaller air bubbles. Hold the syringe upright and pull the plunger back another 0.2 mL (to clear the hub). Then carefully push the plunger up to remove the air. Make sure that the desired amount is left in the syringe. This manipulation can be performed only in a closed system, which means with the cap on the needle.

Using Transfer Needles

Transfer needles are double ended, which means that they have needles on both ends. Transfer needles are useful when the entire contents of a vial are going to be transferred into an IVPB. For example, if you have a vial of Rocephin 1 g IVPB, the entire gram of Rocephin will be reconstituted and added to an IVPB.

To use a transfer needle (Figure 5-6), swab the appropriate areas and place the longer of the two ends in the additive port of the IVPB. Place the shorter end in the desired vial. The transfer needle connects the bag and the vial, allowing the fluid to

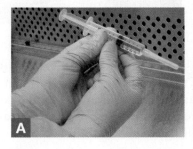
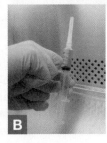
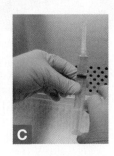

FIGURE 5-5 Removing air bubble

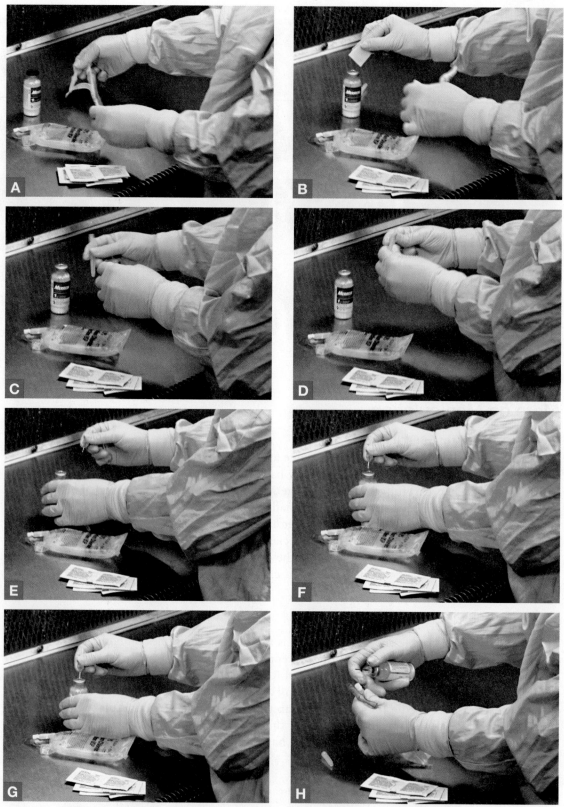

FIGURE 5-6 Using a transfer needle

flow between them. Gently squeeze the IV bag, and the IV fluid will slowly fill the vial. Shake the vial gently until all of the powder is dissolved. When all the powder is dissolved, hold the IV bag so that all of the air floats to the top, then gently squeeze the bag. This process will cause the air to move into the vial, thus creating pressure in the vial. The pressure will force the fluid down into the bag. Since the

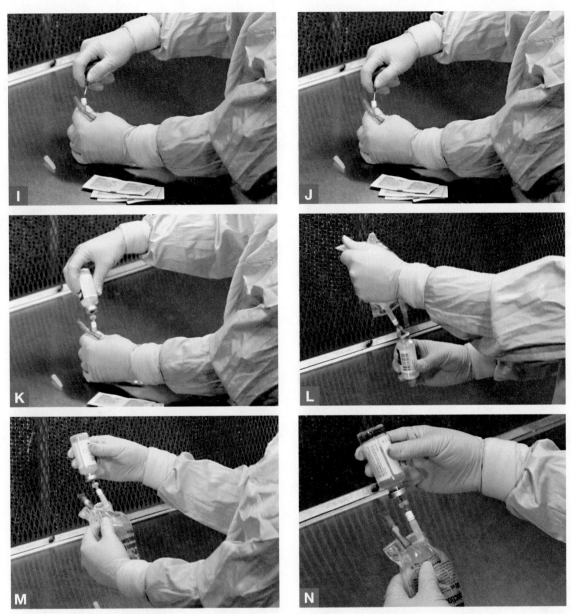

FIGURE 5-6 Using a transfer needle (continued)

addition of Add-A-Vials and Advantage vials, transfer needles are not being used as often as they once were.

Using Ampules

Unlike vials, ampules are composed entirely of glass. After an ampule is opened, it becomes an open system and a single-use container. Because the ampule is an open system (air can pass freely into and out of the ampule), the volume of the fluid removed does not have to be replaced with air. Before an ampule is opened, all of the fluid must be moved from the head and neck (top part) to the body (lower part). This can be accomplished by one of the following methods: swirling the ampule in an upright motion, tapping the head of the ampule with a finger, or inverting the ampule and then quickly swinging it to an upright position. Sometimes one of these methods may be used, and sometimes all three of these methods may be used.

To open an ampule properly, swab the neck of the ampule with alcohol and allow the alcohol to dry. Place a clean alcohol swab on the neck of the ampule. This swab can help prevent accidental cuts to the finger as well as minimize the spraying of glass particles and aerosolized drug. Place the head of the ampule between the thumb and the index finger on one hand, and hold the body of the ampule by the thumb and index finger of the other hand. If the ampule has a dot or line, this indicates a weak area on the neck of the ampule. Exert pressure on both thumbs, pushing the ampule away from yourself in a quick snapping motion. This pressure should cause the neck of the ampule to break (Figure 5-7).

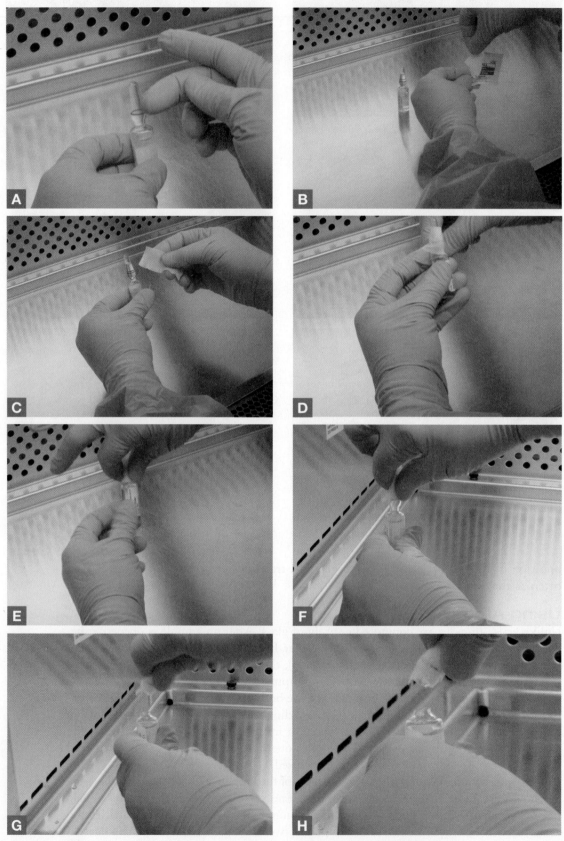

FIGURE 5-7 Opening an ampule

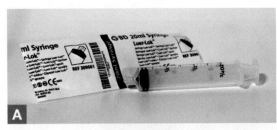

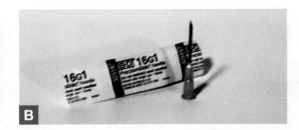

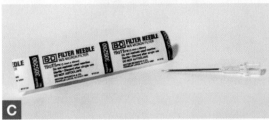

FIGURE 5-8 Filtration methods

Open ampules only to the side of the PEC and never toward the HEPA filter. If an ampule is broken toward the HEPA, small glass particles can damage the filter. Extreme pressure may crush the ampule, but if the ampule does not break easily, rotate the ampule so that the pressure on the neck of the ampule is at a different angle.

To withdraw fluid from the ampule, tilt the ampule downward slightly so that you can place the bevel of a needle in the inside bottom corner of the ampule. Once the fluid covers the bevel of the needle, pull back on the syringe's plunger to withdraw the solution. Since glass particles may have entered the solution as you broke the ampule, you must filter the solution before adding it to a bag. There are several ways to do this (Figure 5-8):

- Draw the medication into a syringe through a filter needle, then change to a regular needle to inject the solution.
- Draw the medication into a syringe through a regular needle, then change to a filter needle to inject the solution.
- Draw the medication up using a filter straw (useful for tall ampules), then change to a regular needle to inject the solution.
- Draw the medication up into a syringe using a regular needle, then push it through an IVEX filter.

Workplace Wisdom

In all cases, do not use the same needle used to withdraw the fluid from the ampule to inject it into an IV bag. A filter needle can be used only once. Using it twice, to withdraw and to inject, will nullify the filtering effort.

PROCEDURE **5-3**

Removing Fluid from an Ampule

You must perform this procedure in the clean air space using proper aseptic technique (Figure 5-9):

1. Follow the proper procedures for dressing and hand washing. Gather all materials needed for the manipulation.
2. Remove any fluid from the neck of the ampule.
3. Swab the neck with alcohol.

(continued)

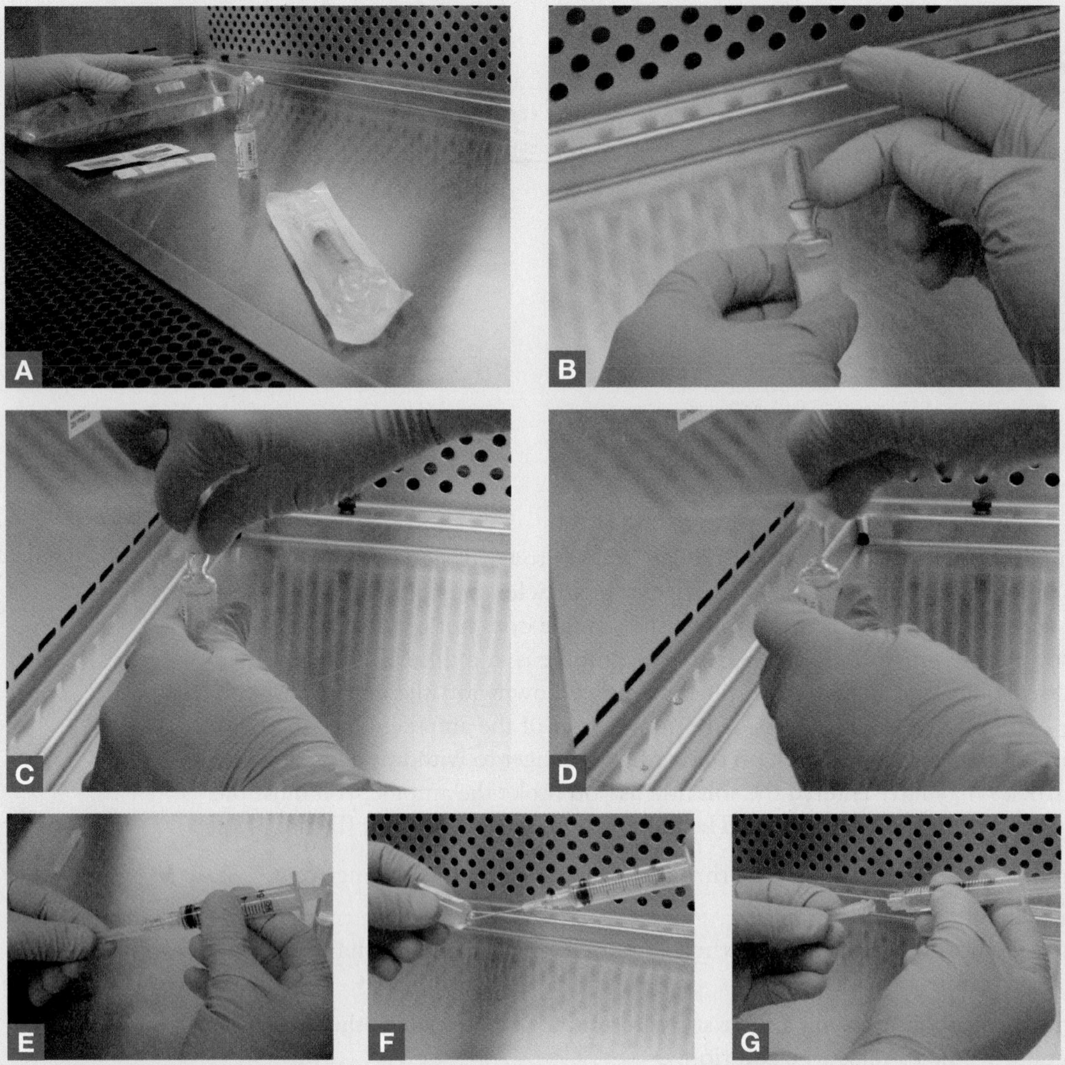

FIGURE 5-9 Withdrawing fluid from an ampule

4. Hold the ampule at a 20-deg angle toward the side of the hood.
5. Using your thumbs, apply pressure toward the neck of the ampule.
6. Using a filter needle, withdraw the fluid.
7. Remove any air bubbles.
8. Change the needle to a regular needle before injecting into a bag.
9. Remove any air bubbles.
10. Insert the needle into the additive port of the IV bag and slowly inject.

Preparing a Sterile Dosage Form

Workplace Wisdom

Never pick up a needle cap in one hand and use it to recap an exposed needle in another hand during the mixing process. Instead, leave the cap on the work surface inside the hood while mixing, then, when ready, slip the needle into the cap and then use the other hand to secure the cap. This prevents unwanted and dangerous needle sticks.

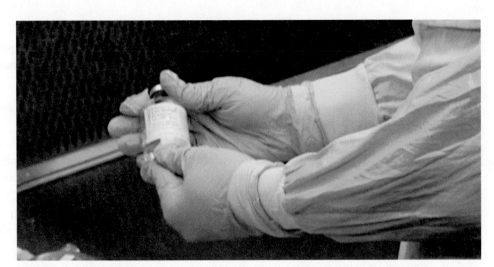

Procedure

Sterile dosage forms may be prepared in various final containers, including flexible plastic bags, glass bottles, glass vials, semirigid plastic containers, and syringes. Before compounding, assemble all materials. Place only necessary materials within the PEC (Figure 5-10).

Next, clean all injection surfaces with a 70% alcohol swab. After the alcohol has dried, withdraw drug fluids aseptically from the containers in the amounts needed, using the appropriate-size syringe. Once all the drug fluids are drawn up, place the syringes with the needles capped on the surface of the hood next to the medication vial. Next to the syringe, place the appropriate base solution. Check the label again to make sure that the correct additives and amounts are drawn up and the correct base is present. Depending on the institutional policy, a pharmacist may be required to check the additives before they are injected into the base. Needles must be carefully inserted into the port of a bag so that the needle does not puncture the bag. If the preparation that is being compounded is a pediatric preparation, a narcotic, a chemotherapy preparation, or a TPN, a pharmacist should check the additives before they are added to the base.

Since large amounts of water and potassium chloride are used during the day, these solutions, attached to transfer tubing, are often hanging in the hood. This enables the technician to draw up large volumes of these solutions very easily. They are easily accessible for stat (urgent or rush) preparations. Large glass bottles (empty evacuated containers) contain a very strong vacuum; therefore, you should never add KCl (potassium chloride) or water to them using a transfer set. The vacuum will continue to draw fluid into the bottle and has the potential to create very dangerous errors in dosing. Therefore, you must draw up SWFI and KCl using individual syringes. Position the injection port of a bag, covered by a protective tip, toward the HEPA filter when preparing an IV admixture, to maintain sterility. If you are using a glass bottle, remove the aluminum cap and place the bottle 6 in. away from the HEPA filter.

Nothing must come between the HEPA filter and the port to which additives are added (this includes vials, syringes, and hands). Disinfect all injection surfaces by swabbing the surface with 70% alcohol and allowing the alcohol to dry. Insert the needle into the rubber stopper or latex diaphragm. Insert needles carefully using a noncoring technique, as described earlier. After you inject the additive, reswab the port with alcohol. Then cover the top of the glass bottle with an IVA seal before removing it from the hood. Once the sterile product is compounded, properly label it and inspect it for cores and particulate matter. If a check has not already been made, place the final solution on the counter with all its contributors and appropriate syringes.

Additional Aseptic Procedures

USP 797 recommends that a pharmacy preparing sterile products adhere to the following standards of practice to help ensure the quality of the compounding area and sterile products.

1. Access to the buffer area must be restricted to qualified personnel assigned to the preparation of sterile products.

2. All supplies in cartons are decontaminated in the area by removing them from shipping cartons and cleaning them with non–residue-generating disinfecting agent while they are being transferred to a clean and properly disinfected cart or other conveyance for introduction into the buffer area.

3. Supplies that are required frequently or otherwise needed close at hand, but not necessarily for scheduled operations, are decontaminated and stored in the anteroom.

4. Carts used to bring supplies from the storeroom cannot be rolled past the demarcation line in the anteroom, and carts used in the buffer area cannot be rolled outward beyond the demarcation line unless they are properly cleaned and disinfected.

5. Generally, supplies required for the scheduled operations of the shift are wiped down with an disinfecting agent and brought into the buffer area, preferably on one or more movable carts. Supplies that are required for backup or general support of operations may be stored on shelving in the buffer area, but excessive stock is to be avoided.

6. Nonessential objects that shed particles should not be brought into the buffer area, including pencils, cardboard, paper towels, and cotton items (e.g., gauge pads).

7. Essential paper-related items (i.e., paper syringe or needle overwraps, work records contained in a protective sleeve) need to be wiped down with a disinfecting agent prior to being introduced into the buffer area.

8. Traffic flow in and out of the buffer area and direct compounding area (DCA) must be minimized and controlled.

9. Personnel entering the buffer area shall remove all personal outer garments, cosmetics (because they shed and flake), and hand, wrist, and other visible jewelry or piercings.

10. Personnel entering the anteroom need to don PPE in the proper order and properly wash hands and forearms up to the elbows for at least 30 sec. Air dryers or lint-free towels are to be used to dry hands and arms.

11. Personnel must perform antiseptic hand cleansing prior to donning sterile gloves, using a waterless, alcohol-based hand scrub with persistent activity.

12. No chewing gum, drinks, candy, or food items will be brought into the ante or buffer areas.

13. At the beginning of each compounding activity session and whenever liquids are spilled, the surfaces of the DCA are first cleaned with purified water to remove water-soluble residues and then immediately disinfected.

14. PECs shall be operated continuously. If blowers are turned off, only one person shall enter the buffer area to turn on the blower (for at least 30 minutes).

15. Supplies used in the DCA for the planned operations are accumulated and then decontaminated by wiping or spraying the outer surface with sterile 70% IPA or removing the out wrap at the edge of the DCA as the item is introduced into the aseptic work area.

16. Arrange all supply items in the DCA to reduce clutter and provide for maximum efficiency and order for the flow of work.

17. Supply items in the DCA should be arranged so that a clear, uninterrupted path of HEPA-filtered air will bathe all critical sites at all times during the procedures. No objects may be placed between the HEPA-filtered air and exposed critical site.

18. All procedures are performed in a manner designed to minimize the risk of touch contamination. Gloves are disinfected with adequate frequency with sterile 70% IPA.

19. Every compounded sterile product must be thoroughly mixed and inspected for the presence of particulate matter, evidence of incompatibility, or other defects.

20. After compounding is complete, used syringes, bottles, vials, and other supplies are removed with a minimum of exit and reentry into the DCA so as to minimize the risk of introducing contamination into the aseptic workspace.

CONCLUSION

You must use proper aseptic technique to prepare a sterile product, free of contaminants, ready for administration. Aseptic technique is a special skill that should become second nature with experience. However, even as you begin to practice aseptic technique, you must strictly follow USP 797 guidelines. If you follow these properly, you will produce a sterile, particulate- and contamination-free product. Following proper protocol helps the preparer avoid potential harm that could occur not only to the patient, but also to the preparer.

PROFILES OF PRACTICE

You are working alone as an IV technician in the IV room. You get three new orders at one time—dopamine for a neonate, Gammar-P IV, and a missing dose for a hydration bag. In what order should you complete these orders and why? (In most institutions, any type of life-saving drug takes precedence.)

DOPAMINE

1. The physician should have specified what he or she would like the dopamine mixed with; if it is not specified, the pharmacist needs to call and clarify. A technician may not take a verbal order. Usually, dopamine is mixed with a dextrose solution.

2. Next, gather the materials needed to withdraw the dopamine and dextrose. Also, remember that since the preparation is for a neonate, all the ingredients must be preservative free, so you need a couple of alcohol swabs and various-size syringes. Remember to be as accurate as possible.

3. Calculate how much dopamine to draw up in a syringe. Using that information, determine how much dextrose you should add to correctly compound the neonatal dopamine.

4. Swab the vials and/or bags and withdraw the correct amounts.

5. Depending on the institution, either call for a pharmacist check or mix the medication and then call for a check. Remember that all items compounded by a technician must be checked.

6. Does the dopamine drip go into a syringe or in an IV bag? Again, you must be familiar with the policies and procedures of the hospital. Of course, this is a *stat* medication, which means that you have about 3 min to make it. What happens if you are wrong?

GAMMAR-P INTRAVENOUS

1. Call the floor and check what time the patient actually needs this medication. This medication is very expensive and has a relatively short expiration time. Conversely, if the nurse needs it now, it takes a while to make.

2. If the nurse needs the Gammar-P IV now, begin swabbing the vials and then reconstitute. While the Gammar-P IV is going into solution, make the hydration bag.

Hydration Bag

a. In order to compound the hydration bag, gather the necessary materials—usually a large-volume IV bag such as NS (normal saline or 0.9% NaCl), KCl (potassium chloride), alcohol swabs, syringes, needles, and "Potassium Added" stickers.

b. Calculate how much KCl you should add to the IV bag.

c. Withdraw the correct amount.

d. Swab the vials and/or bags and withdraw the correct amounts.

e. Depending on the institution, either call for a pharmacist check or mix the medication and then call for a check. Remember that all items compounded by a technician must be checked.

f. Correctly label the bag. Have the pharmacist sign the label, and deliver the IV bag to the floor.

3. Back to the Gammar-P IV, which is still going into solution: You might decide to help the Gammar-P IV and pick up the vial to shake it. However, before you shake the vial, remember that Gammar-P IV is a protein, and protein cannot be shaken. Shaking a protein can damage it. Instead, swirl the vial.

4. When the Gammar-P IV finally goes into solution, carefully transfer all 875 mL of the Gammar-P IV into an empty bag. Call for a check, label the Gammar-P, and deliver it to the floor. You are finally finished with the three new orders and can go back to finishing the regular IV pick.

This scenario could be a common occurrence at a large hospital on any given day. Can you see how any IV technician must possess proficient knowledge in such areas as medical terminology, IV room materials and supplies, different mathematical calculations, and quality assurance? There were only three orders; however, a pharmacy technician must have not only good aseptic skills, but also the knowledge needed to compound these medications correctly.

CHAPTER TERMS

immunocompromised a condition in which the immune system is not functioning normally

reconstitute to add a diluent to a vial to create a liquid

CHAPTER REVIEW QUESTIONS

MULTIPLE CHOICE

1. Dressing mostly takes place in the _____.
   a. anteroom
   b. buffer area
   c. DCA
   d. PEC
   e. bathroom

2. Disposable shoe covers, jackets, face masks, paper arm guards, and facial hair masks are examples of _____.
   a. TPN
   b. CAI
   c. PPE
   d. PEC
   e. DCA

3. All compounding must be performed at least _____ inside the edges of the PEC.
   a. 2 ft
   b. 8 in.
   c. 11 in.
   d. 6 in.
   e. 1 ft

4. If the PEC has been turned off, how long must it be turned on before it can be used? _____
   a. 30 min
   b. 15 min
   c. 60 min
   d. 20 min
   e. 10 min

5. Ampules are made of _____.
   a. plastic
   b. steel
   c. polyurethane
   d. cardboard
   e. glass

6. The process of adding diluent to a powder to form a liquid is known as _____.
   a. manipulating
   b. levigation
   c. reconstitution
   d. emulsifying
   e. additive blending

7. When withdrawing contents from an ampule, what must be used? _____
   a. lint-free towels or gauze
   b. filters
   c. 3-cc syringes
   d. transfer kit
   e. Advantage vial

8. According to American Society of Health-System Pharmacists guidelines, the total volume being measured must be at least _____ of the total size of the syringe.
   a. 20%
   b. 30%
   c. 40%
   d. 15%
   e. 50%

9. After swabbing with alcohol, you must wait for _____ before proceeding when preparing to withdraw contents from a container with a needle/syringe.

   a. the tops to be removed from all the vials of ingredients
   b. the blower in the hood to run for at least 10 min
   c. the pharmacy technician to dress
   d. the alcohol to dry completely
   e. the IV bags to be unwrapped

10. What must you do to all vials before you bring them into the hood?

   a. Remove the tops.
   b. Date them.
   c. Remove the labels.
   d. Stir them slightly to loosen the contents.
   e. Heat them to a lukewarm temperature.

11. A primary engineering control is an ISO Class _____ environment.

   a. 2
   b. 3
   c. 5
   d. 7
   e. 8

12. An anteroom must be an ISO Class _____ or better environment.

   a. 2
   b. 3
   c. 5
   d. 7
   e. 8

13. Hand washing should be performed after putting on the disposable gown.

   a. true
   b. false

14. The PEC should be cleaned with IPA 70% first, then rinsed with sterile water.

   a. true
   b. false

15. Technicians should put on nonsterile gloves prior to entering the buffer area.

   a. true
   b. false

16. Which of the following PPE should be donned first?

   a. face mask
   b. hair cover
   c. gown
   d. shoe covers

17. Protective outer wraps for IV solutions should be removed inside the DCA.

   a. true
   b. false

18. Cosmetics can be worn in the compounding areas as long as they are not applied heavily.

   a. true
   b. false

19. A technician is assigned to prepare sterile products all week long. According to USP guidelines, he or she is allowed to store the materials needed for the entire week in the buffer area.

   a. true
   b. false

20. The technician should always wipe down syringe wrappers before introducing them into the buffer area.

   a. true
   b. false

LABORATORY ACTIVITIES

1. Supplies needed: Shoe covers, head and facial hair covers, mask, soap, lint-free towels, gown, waterless, alcohol-based hand scrub, and sterile, powder-free gloves.

   With these supplies, practice USP 797 gowning, hand washing, and ungowning procedures. Describe them here.

   _____

   _____

   _____

   _____

   _____

2. Supplies needed: liquid 20-mL vial (1); ampule 2 mL (2); ampule 5 mL (1); 10-mL (1), 5-mL (2), and 3-mL (3) syringes; needles (6); filter needles (3); and alcohol swabs. After proper gowning and aseptic hand washing, gather the proper supplies and aseptically withdraw the following dose volumes from the noted vial or ampule one at a time. Remember to maintain aseptic technique and prepare one dose at a time to prevent errors.

MEDICATION	DOSE VOLUME
Liquid 20-mL vial	10 mL
Liquid 20-mL vial	2.5 mL
Liquid 20-mL vial	4.8 mL
Ampule 2 mL	2 mL
Ampule 2 mL	1.4 mL
Ampule 5 mL	4.6 mL

3. Using proper aseptic technique, prepare one dose of each of the following medication orders:
   a. Heparin 1500 units IVP
   b. Heparin 5000 units IV
   c. Tuberculosis skin test 5 tuberculin units
   d. Regular insulin 46 units
   e. Heparin 3000 units IV
   f. Regular insulin 57 units

4. Using proper aseptic technique, prepare one dose of each of the following. Your instructor will provide you with an IV bag to inject the dose into.
   a. Powder Y 1 g IVPB q6h
   b. Powder C 500 mg IVPB q12h
   c. Powder Y 750 mg IVPB BID
   d. Powder C 250 mg IM q8h
   e. Powder Y 0.5 g IVPB q24h
   f. Powder C 250 mg IM q24h

Sterile Product Preparations

6 chapter

After completing this chapter, you should be able to:

- List and describe the different types of sterile products.
- Identify the different uses for large-volume and small-volume IV bags.
- Understand the concept of pediatric dosing and realize why sterile products prepared for this type of patient are different from those for adults.
- List some specialty protein-based sterile products.

Introduction

There are many different ways to prepare sterile products for administration. Some medications are aseptically compounded into a syringe or into a large-volume or small-volume IV bag, and some may be in the form of irrigations or ophthalmic solutions. All pharmacy-prepared sterile products should be compounded in a primary engineering control such as a laminar airflow hood (LAH), biological safety cabinet (BSC), or compounding aseptic isolator (CAI). This chapter will explore the different ways that sterile products can be packaged for proper administration.

Intravenous Bags

The most common type of sterile product is the IV bag. IV bags contain base solutions to which medication is then added and diluted before administration. For example, if Fortaz (an antibiotic) is administered IV without being diluted, it will cause a severe burning sensation to the patient. Other medications, such as potassium chloride (KCl), can cause death when undiluted.

IV bags can be classified into one of two main categories. IV bags that are administered on an intermittent or on a specific schedule, such as twice daily or three times a day, are referred to as **intravenous piggybacks (IVPB)** (Figures 6-1 and 6-2). The second group of IVs, large-volume IVs or drips, are infused on a continuous basis over longer periods of time.

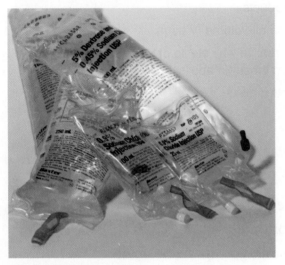

FIGURE 6-1 Intravenous bags

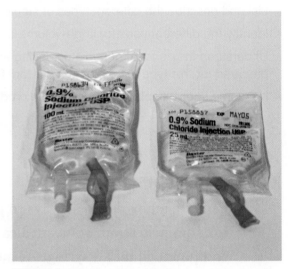

FIGURE 6-2   Intravenous piggyback

Intravenous Piggybacks

Intravenous piggybacks or small-volume parenterals (SVP) are administered over a short period of time at specific intervals. They also usually have a smaller volume than a continuous infusion. These IVs consist of a base fluid, usually D5W or NS, and a medication additive. In general, most IVPB base solutions range in volume from 25 to 250 mL.

The objective of the IVPB is to administer a medication that (a) the patient cannot take via another method or (b) needs to act quickly. These IVs are usually some type of antibiotic, antifungal, antiviral, mineral replacement, or maintenance medication. Antibiotics include, but are not limited to, Unasyn, Claforan, Fortaz, vancomycin, and Zosyn. Antivirals include, but are not limited to, Zovirax and Cytovene. Mineral replacements may include potassium chloride, sodium chloride, and calcium gluconate. Maintenance medication includes Dilantin, valproic acid, and Cerebyx.

Medications used to make IVPBs are available from the manufacturer in either a solution or a powder that must be reconstituted before being added to the base solution. IVPBs that are manually prepared by aseptically transferring medication from one container to another have shorter shelf lives.

Another option for manual IVPB preparation is the use of Add-a-Vial or Advantage systems. These systems allow the medication vial to be attached aseptically to the base solution without actually mixing the drug with the solution. The drug is mixed into the solution by the caregiver shortly before administration to the patient. The advantage to these types of systems is that the IVPBs have a longer expiration date than manually prepared sterile products.

Table 6-1 Infusion Fluid Abbreviations

¼NS	0.22% Sodium chloride
½NS	0.45% Sodium chloride
BWFI	Bacteriostatic water for injection
D5W	Dextrose 5% in water (5% dextrose injection, USP)
D10W	Dextrose 10% in water (10% dextrose injection, USP)
D20W	Dextrose 20% in water (20% dextrose injection, USP)
D5LR	Dextrose in lactated Ringer's solution (5% dextrose in lactated Ringer's injection)
D5 ¼NS	Dextrose 5% in quarter-strength saline (5% dextrose and 0.22% sodium chloride injection, USP)
D5 ½NS	Dextrose 5% in half-strength saline (5% dextrose and 0.45% sodium chloride injection, USP)
D5NS	Dextrose 5% in normal saline (5% dextrose and 0.9% sodium chloride injection, USP)
D5R	Dextrose 5% in Ringer's injection (5% dextrose in Ringer's injection)
D10NS	Dextrose 10% in normal saline (10% dextrose and 0.9% sodium chloride injection, USP)
IS10W	Invert sugar 10% in saline (10% invert sugar in 0.9% sodium chloride injection)
LR	Lactated Ringer's injection, USP
Pr	Protein hydrolysate (protein hydrolysate injection, USP)
NS	Sodium chloride 0.9% (normal saline) (0.9% sodium chloride injection, USP)
SWFI	Sterile water for injection

A number of IVPBs come from manufacturers premade, and some need to be kept frozen until use. Antibiotics are the primary type of frozen IVPBs. The advantage of premade IVPBs is that, if stored properly, they remain sterile and effective until their printed expiration date. However, if the premixed IVPBs are removed from their over-wraps or if they are defrosted, their expiration will significantly shorten. Premixed IVPBs do not require an aseptic environment, only proper labeling and a final check by a pharmacist before delivery to the patient.

Continuous Preparations

Large-Volume Intravenous Bags and Large-Volume Parenterals

Most large-volume IV (LVIV) bags (Figure 6-3) are infused on a continuous rate and are mainly used for hydration and electrolyte/vitamin replacement. Large-volume IVs are generally 500 mL or greater, with the most common size being 1 L (1000 mL). Many large-volume parenterals (LVPs) may consist only of a base solution with no additives. However, if needed, the most common additives are electrolytes and vitamins, as they can also be depleted when a patient is dehydrated. Large volumes can also be continuous antibiotic infusions, which are sometimes necessary to treat severe infections.

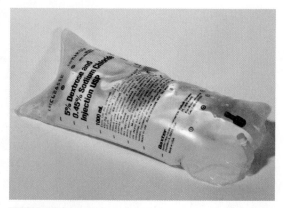

FIGURE 6-3 Large-volume bag

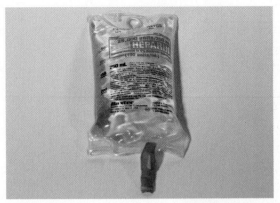

FIGURE 6-4 Drip

Drips

Drips (Figure 6-4) are usually infused at a very slow rate and contain medications other than electrolytes or vitamins. Most drips are 500 mL or less; they often contain drugs such as nitroglycerin, insulin, amiodarone, lidocaine, nitroprusside, heparin, and narcotics. Prescribers order drips by the amount of drug to be infused over a given time frame (mg/kg per min or mcg/hr). Hospitals have specific policies and procedures that deal with these medications because they are very specific and can be costly to make.

Syringes

To give an IVP, syringes are the dosage form used (Figure 6-5). Some IVP medications, such as skin tests, vaccinations, and colony-stimulating factors, can be given without being diluted, whereas others, such as patient-controlled analgesia and pediatric and neonatal antibiotics, are diluted.

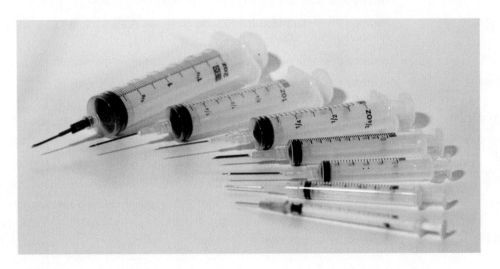

FIGURE 6-5 Syringes

Multidose Vials

A multidose vial (MDV) is one that is designed to be used more than one time for more than one dose of medication. MDVs (Figure 6-6) are designed to retain sterility after more than one needle puncture and usually contain preservatives. If a MDV is used for

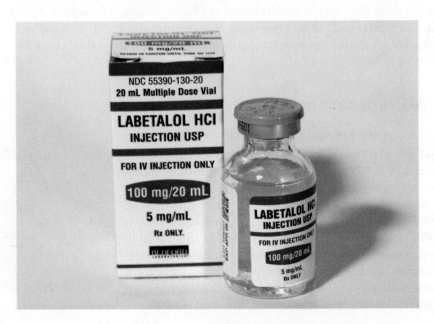

FIGURE 6-6 Multidose vial

a dose, the remainder in the vial must be stored properly and used before the expiration date. The person opening a MDV must write the date and time opened and his or her initials on the vial. The expiration date or beyond-use date for a MDV is 28 days unless otherwise specified by the drug manufacturer.

Patient-Controlled Analgesia

Patient-controlled analgesia (PCA) (Figure 6-7) is an IV pain medication in which the patient controls the delivery of the drug. When the patient begins to have pain, he or she has a button to push to receive a dose of pain medication through the IV line. PCA is administered through various types of IV pumps and devices. Although the patient determines when he or she receives the medication, all PCA devices are calibrated to "lock" the patient out so that he or she does not overdose.

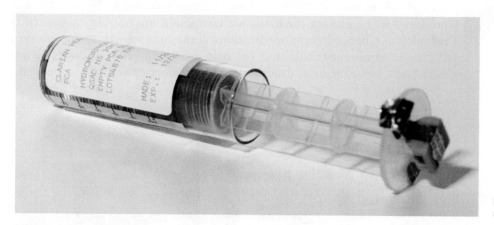

FIGURE 6-7 Patient-controlled anesthesia

Epidurals

Epidurals are inserted intrathecally and are used to help control pain in conjunction with surgery or obstetrics (Figure 6-8). Epidurals may consist of a narcotic and an anesthetic, such as bupivacaine or ropivacaine, or just an anesthetic, depending on the patient's needs. The important thing to remember about compounding epidurals is that all medication must be preservative free. The most common preservative, benzyl alcohol, can cause paralysis if used in an epidural.

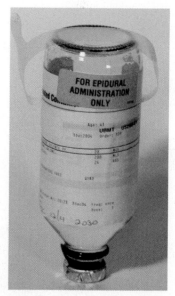

FIGURE 6-8 Epidural

Neonates and Pediatric Patients

Most of the time, dilutions are used for neonates and pediatric patients. Dilutions are a way to take a more concentrated substance and make it less concentrated and are usually used when a dose is so small that it cannot be measured accurately. For example, insulin comes as 100 units/mL, and a neonate dose may be 5 units. Without diluting the insulin, the measurement would 0.05 mL, which is a very minute amount in the syringe. With very small measurements, it is easy to unintentionally draw up an inaccurate dose. However, if the insulin is diluted from 100 to 10 units/mL, then the same 5-unit dose is now 0.5 mL, which is much easier to accurately measure and administer.

The other reason for using dilutions is that the organ systems of neonatal and pediatric patients are still developing. Their liver and kidneys do not metabolize and excrete medications as efficiently as those of most adults. Diluting the medication, or putting the dose in a larger fluid amount, is less taxing on the developing systems. Medications that can be made into a dilution include, but are not limited to, antibiotics, antifungals, antivirals, narcotics, and insulin.

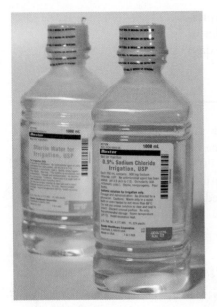

FIGURE 6-9 Irrigation

Irrigations

Two of the most common sterile **irrigations** (Figure 6-9) are surgical antibiotic solution and gentamicin irrigation solution. Although they are not infused intravenously, irrigations must be compounded in a sterile environment, as they typically are used in surgery to irrigate open surgical sites. The sterile water or normal saline to which Neosporin and gentamicin are added are sterile and are labeled "For Irrigation Only," which indicates that the solutions are sterile but do not meet the requirements for intravenous use.

Cytotoxic Agents

Cytotoxic (chemotherapy) medications (Figure 6-10) are always compounded in a BSC. The BSC has a different direction of airflow (vertical) that allows the IV technician to compound cytotoxic medications more safely. Instead of flowing toward the IV technician, the air is blown vertically down; in this way, the aerosols produced when making the cytotoxic compound are not blown toward the IV technician. Chemotherapy medications come in a variety of forms: syringes, IVPBs, or continuous infusions. The only difference between cytotoxic medications and other dangerous drugs is where they are aseptically compounded.

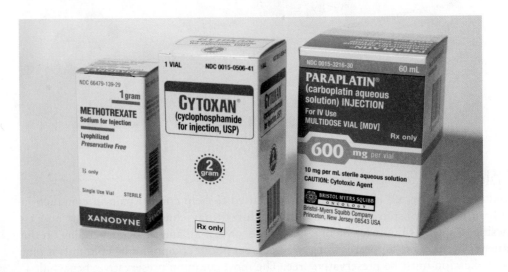

FIGURE 6-10 Cytotoxic agents

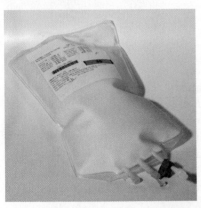

FIGURE 6-11 Total parenteral nutrition bag

Total Parenteral Nutrition

A physician may decide to order a total parenteral nutrition (TPN) bag (Figure 6-11) if a patient has not been able to receive adequate nutrition via other means. TPNs provide the patient with all their dietary requirements to sustain life; they contain protein, fat, sugar, water, minerals, electrolytes, and vitamins. TPNs are compounded daily, usually every 24 hours, specific to the patient's needs and size, and may range in IV bag size from 500 to 3000 mL.

Proteins

Special preparations are also an important part of the aseptic compounding in an IV room. Most of these special preparations are proteins. They should never be filtered, as they will stick to the filter, thus altering the dose given.

Albumin

Some special preparations are albumin, plasma protein fraction, Gammar-P, factor VIII, and factor IX. Albumin is a sterile solution for a single-dose administration, containing 25% human albumin. Albumin is used to treat hypovolemic shock, in conjunction with exchange transfusion, in the treatment of neonatal hyperbilirubinemia and for other conditions. Albumin may be a floor stock item in critical care areas. Do not use albumin solutions if they appear turbid or if there is sediment in the bottle. Begin administration within 4 hours after the bottle is punctured. Dispose of empty albumin vials in an approved sharps container.

Plasma Protein Fraction

Plasma protein fraction (PPF) is a sterile solution for single-dose intravenous administration containing 5% plasma proteins. PPF is used to prevent and treat hypovolemic shock and cases of severe hypoproteinuria, as in adjunct hemodialysis. Do not use solutions of PPF if they appear turbid or if there is sediment in the bottle. Begin administration within 4 hours after the container has been entered. Dispose of empty PPF vials in an approved sharps container.

Immunoglobulin

Immune globulin (Gammar-P, IgG) intravenous is a sterile, lyophilized, single-dose preparation of immune globulin. Gammar-P is indicated for patients with primary defective or suppressed immune systems, who are at increased risk of infection. Wear chemo gloves when preparing this product. Do not mix immune globulin products of differing formulations.

IgG must be reconstituted before being administered. Most IgG preparations include a double-ended, vented spike adapter with a plastic piercing pin, and it is very important to use the transfer pins correctly. Failure to follow the reconstitution instructions could lead to contamination of the product and/or loss of vacuum, which would the make the IgG impossible to reconstitute. Read the package insert for step-by-step reconstitution instructions. Do not shake the product vial, as excessive foaming and protein bruising will occur. Gently swirl the vial once the diluent has been added. Use within 24 hours of reconstitution or as recommended by the package insert. Visually inspect the solution for any particulate matter and discoloration prior to administration. Dispose of empty IgG containers, tubings, and so on in an approved sharps container. Check with the pharmacy's policies and procedures before compounding any IgG, as Gammar-P has a short stability time and is very expensive.

Factor VIII

Factor VIII (Alphanate) is a sterile, lyophilized, single-dose concentrate of antihemophilic factor (AHF). Factor VIII is used to prevent and control bleeding in patients with factor VIII deficiency due to hemophilia A or acquired factor VIII deficiency. Wear chemo gloves when preparing this product. Do not mix factor VIII products from differing formulations.

Ordered by international units, lyophilized factor VIII concentrate is available in many different sizes. The number of units in the vial varies with each lot number.

Because factor VIII is stored in the refrigerator, it must be warmed to room temperature, as this will facilitate the concentrate's dissolution. Reconstitute exactly as according to the package insert instructions. Gently swirl the contents once the diluent has been added, but do not shake the reconstituted product, as excessive foaming will result. Withdraw the reconstituted product into a syringe through the vented filter spike provided in the package, and do not fill the syringe to more than two thirds of its maximum capacity.

Before capping with a red Luer-lock syringe cap, draw approximately 10 cc of air into the syringe. This will reduce bubbling and foaming and, more important, will reduce the risk of exposure to nursing staff if the AHF leaks into the cap or the transport bag. Administer factor VIII within 8 hours or as directed in the package insert. Discard all empty AHF vials and associated tubing, equipment, and so on into an approved sharps container.

Check with the pharmacy's policies and procedures before compounding any scheduled doses of factor VIII since this product has a short stability, is extremely expensive, and is very unlikely to be able to be used on another patient.

Factor IX

Factor IX (Konyne) is a sterile, lyophilized, single-dose concentrate of AHF intended for IV administration to treat factor IX deficiency. The reconstitution, handling, delivery, and other procedures used when working with factor IX are exactly the same as described previously for factor VIII. For more detailed information, consult the package insert or other approved literature (Figure 6-12).

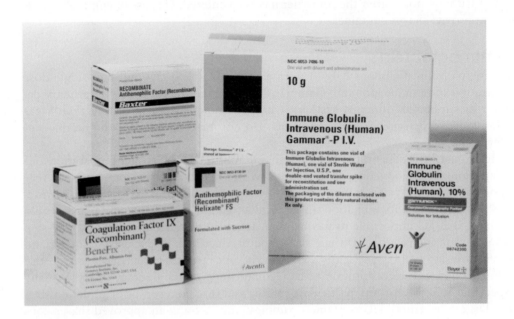

FIGURE 6-12 Special protein products

Ophthalmics

Ophthalmics are also prepared using proper aseptic technique (Figure 6-13). Although most ophthalmic preparations are available from a manufacturer, special strengths or formulations that must be compounded by the pharmacy may be prescribed. Compounded preparations are sterilized by filtration before being packaged into the ophthalmic dropper bottle.

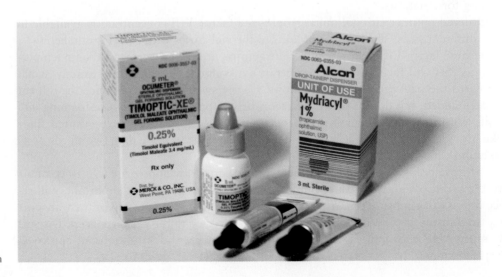

FIGURE 6-13 Ophthalmic preparation

CONCLUSION

A wide variety of dosage forms are used in conjunction with sterile products, depending on the desired route of administration. The most common route of administration that requires aseptic preparation is intravenous. The IV route of administration involves a large number of potential dosage forms, including syringes, IVPBs, drips, and large-volume IV bags. With experience you will learn not only how a specific product is made, but also the best method of preparation.

CHAPTER TERMS

intravenous piggyback (IVPB) a small-volume IV fluid that normally has medication added

irrigation a solution used for washing

CHAPTER REVIEW QUESTIONS

MULTIPLE CHOICE

1. Which is the most common dosage form for IV administration?
   a. syringes
   b. IV bags
   c. epidurals
   d. ophthalmics

2. What is the most common way that IV antibiotics are infused?
   a. large volumes
   b. syringes
   c. intravenous piggybacks
   d. irrigations

3. A TB skin test would be administered via _____.
   a. syringe
   b. IVPB
   c. LVP
   d. none of the above

4. A physician writes an order for IV dopamine. This would most likely be compounded as a _____.
   a. syringe
   b. IVPB
   c. drip
   d. intrathecal

5. A 1-L bag of D5NS infused at 125 mL/hr is considered a _____.
   a. syringe
   b. IVPB
   c. continuous infusion
   d. SVP

6. A physician writes an order for an epidural that has fentanyl and bupivacaine in normal saline. Which of the following statements is incorrect?
   a. The IV technician should take into account the total size of the epidural.
   b. The IV technician should never put narcotics in an epidural.
   c. The IV technician should never put preservatives in an epidural.
   d. The IV technician must use aseptic technique.

7. A _____ vial allows the medication in the IV bag to be mixed just before administration.
   a. last-minute-adding
   b. Micromix
   c. Advantage
   d. epidural
   e. none of the above

8. PCA stands for _____.
   a. patient comfort anesthesia
   b. piggyback chemical additives
   c. partially combined additives
   d. piggyback combined analgesia
   e. patient-controlled analgesia

9. Surgical antibiotic solution (SAS) is an example of a sterile compounded _____.
   a. irrigation
   b. epidural
   c. PCA
   d. IV piggyback
   e. drip

10. PCA cannot contain preservatives.
    a. true
    b. false

LABORATORY ACTIVITIES

1. Determine if the following would be an IVPB, LVP, or drip.

   a. D5 ½NS with 20 KCl/L @ 50 mL/hr

   _____

   b. Cefazolin 1 g in 50 mL D5W

   _____

   c. Nitroglycerin 50 mg in 500 mL

   _____

   d. NS 1 L w/1000 mcg B12

   _____

   e. Diphenhydramine 50 mg/100 mL NS

   _____

   f. Heparin 20,000 units/500 mL NS

   _____

2. You have a pediatric patient who requires Regular insulin. You need to dilute the stock concentration of 100 units/mL to 10 units/mL. Using proper aseptic technique, prepare 10 mL of Regular insulin 10 units/mL. Describe what you did.

   _____

   _____

   _____

   _____

   _____

   _____

   _____

   _____

Total Parenteral Nutrition

After completing this chapter, you should be able to:

- Explain why a patient receives a TPN.
- List the additives used in making a TPN.
- Explain why the ingredients are necessary in a TPN.
- Describe how to admix a TPN.
- Discuss automated mixing equipment.

Introduction

Total parenteral nutrition (TPN) provides needed daily nutritional requirements to a patient with severe gastrointestinal distress and/or poor nutrient absorption. TPNs are given to patients who cannot or should not receive their nutrition through the gastrointestinal tract and are prescribed by a physician to meet that patient's entire nutritional needs. TPNs nourish the body and relieve the digestive tract while therapy for the underlying condition progresses.

TPN, also known as hyperalimentation or hyperals, contains protein, lipids, sugar, electrolytes, vitamins, and other essential elements. This liquid food nutrition is infused directly into a central vein, with the IV bags typically running over a 24 hour period.

TPN is indicated in patients with the following conditions:

- cancer
- AIDS
- Crohn's disease
- surgical removal of the intestines
- severe diarrhea
- hyperemesis gravidarum (uncontrollable vomiting during pregnancy)
- premature **neonate**
- coma

The Ingredients

TPNs have many different components and may have up to 15 to 20 additives, which makes them extremely complex sterile compounds. Therefore, the more complex they are, the higher is the incidence of error or incompatibility. A common TPN bag volume is between 500 mL and 4 L, with the average adult patient receiving 3–4 L/day. Maintaining aseptic technique when preparing TPNs is essential, as they provide a fertile medium for the growth of microorganisms.

The components of a TPN can be classified as either a base solution or an additive. The base solution includes the following:

- **Dextrose**—a source of carbohydrates or sugar used to provide the patient with calories and energy
- **Amino Acids**—a source of protein used to build, maintain, and replace body tissues
- **Lipids**—a source of fat used to provide calories and energy storage
- **Sterile Water**—used to adjust the volume of the TPN

TPN additives include the following:

- **Electrolytes**—such as sodium, potassium, chloride, phosphate, calcium, and magnesium
- **Trace elements**—such as zinc, copper, manganese, and chromium
- **Vitamins**

A TPN order may contain all or some of these substances, depending on the patient's condition. Everyone needs these base ingredients in addition to other substances to stay healthy.

Fluid Maintenance

The physician will begin by deciding the total volume of the TPN and choosing the base fluids. A first estimate of maintenance fluid requirements can be obtained from body weight or from body surface area. The figure based on body weight is obtained from the following formula:

Total fluid requirement = 100 mL/kg for the first 10 kg of body weight

+ 50 mL/kg for the next 10 kg of body weight

+ 20 mL/kg for each additional kilogram above 20 kg

Factors that can affect these amounts include dehydration, overhydration, and related conditions. Patients are monitored for fluid balance variations as well as nutritional needs.

Calories and Carbohydrates

The most common sources of calories and carbohydrates are dextrose and lipids. Dextrose is available in a wide range of concentrations, from 2.5% to 70%, with 50% and 70% being the most common strength used for TPN admixtures. Each gram of dextrose provides 3.45 kcal (kilocalories).

Lipids are added to prevent essential fatty acid deficiency and in combination with dextrose to contribute to the total caloric content. Lipids are available in concentrations of 10%, 20%, and 30%. The 10% or 20% concentrations may be infused directly into the vein, while the 30% concentration must be mixed into the TPN bag because the osmolarity and pH balance of body fluids are more compatible with the 10% and 20% concentrations than with the 30% concentration. It is estimated that an average healthy patient's caloric support is best provided as a mixed fuel, with 50%–80% of the calories derived from dextrose and 20%–50% from fat. Each gram of fat provides approximately 9 kcal.

Amino Acids

Amino acids are the molecular units that make up proteins and are considered the building blocks of the body because they build, maintain, and repair body tissues. Eight of the 22 standard amino acids are considered essential because they are not produced by the body. The remaining are considered nonessential amino acids because the body has the ability to synthesize them. Amino acids also provide the body with nitrogen, which aids in protein metabolism. Nitrogen levels need to be monitored and maintained, and they can vary based on different stress situations with the patient.

Electrolytes and Minerals

The physician prescribes the required amount of electrolytes and minerals based on the patient's needs determined through lab testing and assessment. It is extremely important that TPN orders continue to be reassessed, as the patient's needs vary daily with therapy. These additives are calculated to provide and maintain a proper balance within the body. The amounts must be accurately determined to prevent metabolic disturbances and other serious health consequences due to one or more deficiencies.

Table 7-1 presents average daily electrolyte and mineral requirements and their function during intravenous feeding. In addition to the ingredients shown in Table 7-1, trace elements (for growth and development), multivitamins, and vitamin K (needed for proper blood coagulation) can be added to the admixture as well. Note that if vitamin K is needed, it is added only one time per week.

The Order

The life cycle of a TPN order begins with the physician. After assessing the patient and determining that a TPN is necessary, a physician will write the order and send it to the pharmacy to be compounded. Most facilities that compound TPN solutions will have written **protocols** for the management of TPN. Patients are assessed daily, and appropriate changes are made based on the clinical course of the patient and available laboratory data.

Table 7-1 Daily Electrolyte and Mineral Requirements

SUBSTANCE	DAILY REQUIREMENT	USE
Sodium	80–100 mEq/day	Determines total body water May be added as chloride, lactate, acetate, or phosphate salt
Potassium	80–100 mEq/day	Contributes to proper nerve and muscle function (including the heart); regulates the water balance of cells; balances electrolytes May be added as chloride, phosphate, or acetate salt
Chloride	Usually equal to sodium	Helps keep the amount of fluid inside and outside cells in balance; helps maintain proper blood volume, blood pressure, and pH of body fluids; to avoid acid–base disturbances due to chloride ion abnormalities, the infused sodium:chloride ratio should be adjusted to 1:1 by using acetate, lactate, or phosphate salts instead of chloride
Calcium	15–20 mEq (0.2–0.3 mEq/ kg per day)	Necessary for many normal functions of the body, especially bone formation and maintenance—nerve function, muscle contraction, blood clotting, and proper heart function; given as gluconate, glucoheptonate, or gluceptate salt
Magnesium	15–25 mEq (0.25–0.35 mEq/ kg per day)	Important for many systems in the body, especially the muscles and nerves; given as magnesium sulfate
Phosphate	20–30 mM (7–9 mM/ 1000 kcal)	Needed for bone growth, energy, fighting infection, and proper muscle function; given as potassium or sodium phosphate

The hospital pharmacy may have a *standard order*, which is the basic, nonspecialized TPN order for an average TPN patient, as part of its protocol, or the physician can deviate from the standard order and create his or her specialized TPN order. An example of a TPN order for a transplant patient can bee seen in Figure 7-1. Each order will consider whether the TPN with a hypertonic mixture of amino acids and a dextrose

---

15246
CH-69
(JUN 02)

013105

ADULT PARENTERAL NUTRITION ORDER

A. Check INDICATION for Parenteral Nutrition

☐ Bowel Ischemia   ☐ Gi Bowel Obstruction/Teus
☐ IDB/short bowel syndrome   ☐ Fistula
☐ Intractable Vomiting/Diarrhea   ☐ Other _____

03/11/1944   F 12/27/04

TRANSPLANT
INPATIENT

B. BASE SOLUTION
☐ **CUSTOM CENTRAL FORMULA**
1. Protein
    Crystalline Amino Acids ___60___ g/days
    Hepatamine* (40 g/bottle) _____ g/days
2. Nonprotein Calories (NPC)
    Dextrose ____1000____ kcal/day
    Fat _____300_____ kcal/day
3. Total volume (check one)
    ☐ a. Maximally concentrated solution
    ☒ b. _____1800_____ mL/day

☐ **STANDARD CENTRAL FORMULA** (per liter)

Amino Acids	50g
Dextrose	600 kcal (175g)
Fat	300 kcal (30g)
Total kcal	1100 kcal/L
Total Volume	_____ mL/day

☐ **STANDARD PERIPHERAL FORMULA** (per liter)

Amino Acids	30g
Dextrose	240 kcal (70g)
Fat	400 kcal (40g)
Total kcal	760 kcal/L
Osmolarity	710 mOsm/L
Total Volume	_____ mL/day

C. ADDITIVES (Guidelines for electrolytes/vitamins on back)

☐ CUSTOM		☐ STANDARD	
Sodium Acetate	__40__ mEq/day	Sodium Phosphate	20 mE/day
Potassium Chloride	__40__ mEq/day	Magnesium Sulfate	12 mEq/day
Potassium Phosphate	_____ mEq/day	Multivitamin	10 mEq/day
Calcium Gluconate	__5__ mEq/day	Insulin (Humulin R)	_____ units/day
Multi-Trace Elements	1 mL/day		

D. METABOLIC MONITORING Check box if desired. (Enter I.U. Order No. in parenthesis.)

☐ Chem 7 qd or q _____   ( )   ☐ Glucose monitoring q 6 hours or q _____   ( )
☐ Ionized Ca. Phos. Mg q. Monday/Thusday   ( )   ☐ Hepatic Panel and Triglycerides q Monday   ( )
☐ Prealbumin every Monday   ( )   ☐ Weigh patient qd or q _____   ( )

Special Instructions: _____

Physician Signature: _____   Date _1/31/05_ Time ___13,30___

RN/Unit Secretary Signature: _____   Date _____ Time _____

WHITE-MED. RECORD CANARY-PHARMACY	**ADULT PARENTERAL NUTRITION ORDERS**							**T-5**
B.-CLIN. NOTES	**E-LAB**	**G-X-RAY**	**K-DIAGNOSTIC**	**M-SURGERY**	**Q-THERAPY**	**T-ORDERS**	**W-NURSING**	**Y-MISC.**

FIGURE 7-1 Total parenteral nutrition order

concentration above 10% must be administered though a **central line,** which can be inserted directly or peripherally. TPN with a dextrose concentration 10% or below can be infused through a **peripheral line.** Factors considered when deciding on a peripheral or central line include the following:

- Type of medication being administered
- Osmolarity and pH of the solution to be infused
- Duration of therapy
- Diagnosis or medical condition of the patient
- Patient preferences
- Current availability and status of patient's veins
- Patient history
- Secondary risk factors

There may be other factors to consider as well. Each patient is assessed as an individual.

It is important to infuse the TPN solution at a steady rate. Large changes can result in significant **hypoglycemia** or **hyperglycemia.** Therefore, a patient beginning TPN therapy must have the infusion rate tapered up over several hours until the desired rate is achieved. Similarly, when TPN therapy is discontinued, the infusion rate must be tapered down until the infusion stops. If the infusion must be interrupted, a bag of low-concentration dextrose, typically 10%, can be infused during the interruption to help prevent sudden hypoglycemia caused by the high endogenous insulin secretion associated with the infusion of hypertonic dextrose.

Compounding the Total Parenteral Nutrition

When the pharmacy receives a TPN order, the pharmacist or pharmacy technician checks the patient's lab values. The pharmacist then compares the lab values to the TPN order and suggests any clinical changes if necessary. The pharmacist also goes over the calcium gluconate and potassium phosphate levels to help ensure that the TPN will not precipitate. Phosphate supplementation is often incompatible with calcium, which causes the formation of an insoluble salt.

After checking the levels, the pharmacist or pharmacy technician performs the calculations necessary to determine how a TPN will physically be made. For example, if the order is written for 6 mEq KCl per liter and the total actual volume (TAV) is 1.5 L, then 9 mEq needs to be added to the TPN ($6 \times 1.5 = 9$). If KCl comes as 2 mEq/mL, this means that 4.5 mL of KCl must be added to the TPN ($\frac{9}{2} = 4.5$). If the pharmacy technician calculates the additive volumes, a pharmacist must double-check them. Some hospitals require two pharmacists to check the TPN calculations before preparing the TPN. It is very easy to make mistakes when dealing with TPNs, as they are very complex. Great detail and care must be exercised.

After the TPN calculations are completed and double-checked, it is time to compound the TPN. TPNs must be compounded in an ISO 5 environment. The base solution is always compounded first. Then the additives are drawn up. After the pharmacist checks the base solutions and the additives, the pharmacy technician can inject the additives into the prepared base.

Carefully check the amounts needed for each ingredient and choose the correct-size bags, syringes, and needles. For example, if 6 mL of a product is needed, then choose the next higher syringe, 10 mL, for drawing up that particular ingredient. To choose a bag, calculate the final volume of the TPN and use a bag in which the entire TPN will fit easily. It is better to choose a bag that is too big than one that is not big enough.

Workplace Wisdom

Check with the hospital's policies and procedures to see if syringes are uniformly placed on the right or left side of the vial. Whatever the pharmacy decides, it should remain consistent to help prevent medication errors. Remember, it is very difficult to determine what is in a clear, unmarked syringe. When in doubt, toss it out.

TPN base solutions can be compounded either using an automated device or manually by the gravity method. When compounding TPN base solutions using the gravity method, the pharmacy technician manually runs all the needed solutions into the empty TPN bag using a transfer IV set. The transfer set is aseptically attached to the base solution bags (dextrose, amino acids, lipids, sterile water) and is hung from the IV pole. The other end of the transfer set is attached to the empty bag, and gravity allows the base solutions to flow into the empty TPN container. A port adapter can be used for multiple injections several times while making only one injection into the TPN bag, ensuring that TPN bag injection port is not compromised.

When using an automated device, add the base components to the empty TPN bag in the following order: dextrose, amino acids, lipids, and SWFI. If compounding by the gravity method, do not add the lipids until all additives have injected because the lipids are opaque white and will prevent visual inspection of precipitates and other particulates in the solution. The amino acids will act as a buffer between the dextrose and lipids to minimize any possible chemical reaction. When the base solution contains lipids, it is called 3-in-1 solution.

After the base solutions are compounded, it is time to begin drawing up the electrolytes, trace elements, and vitamins into individual syringes. After you withdraw the additives, place the syringes to the right of the vial from which they were withdrawn. Because most TPNs have multiple additives, the space in your DCA can become constricted, causing errors in aseptic technique to occur.

After you draw up the additives, the pharmacist must perform a final check. After the final check is complete, inject the additive syringes into the TPN bag. When injecting additives to a TPN, do so in the following order:

1. Any electrolye containing phosphate
2. All other additives (except calcium and multivitamin)
3. Any electrolyte containing calcium
4. Multivitamin and/or any additive with color

Make sure to gently mix the bag in between each addition of the additives. This mixing is critical, especially between the additions of the phosphate and calcium. Mixing phosphate and calcium together or closely together can cause precipitation to occur in a TPN. After the calcium is injected and before adding the multivitamin (MVI) or color, be sure to visually check the TPN bag for any incompatibilities or precipitation. The MVI is added last so that any precipitation is not masked by its color. If you add any proteins such as insulin or albumin to the TPN, do not use filters to inject the dose into the TPN bag, as the proteins will stick to the filters, altering the dose. When you have finished admixing all ingredients, gently shake or rotate the bag to blend and distribute the ingredients evenly.

If the TPN has been compounded manually, it will be time to add the lipids. Lipids form a solid, milky white liquid and are added last because they will mask any particulate or precipitation in the final solution. This is why some institutions will not mix lipids directly into the TPN bag and infuse lipids as an IVPB in conjunction with the TPN.

When you add the calcium and again when you have finished adding all ingredients, be certain to carefully visually inspect the solution and take time to closely survey and notice any particulates. If you find any, notify the pharmacist immediately.

Before delivering the solution to the patient, some facilities will include an inline filter. There is some debate over the usefulness of such filters and whether they are necessary. One concern is that they may clog the additives, such as the fat emulsions. Check with the facility and its procedures to see if a filter is included with TPN solutions.

It is extremely important for the pharmacy technician to learn what supplies are available for compounding and what procedures are followed. Some supplies make compounding easier, reducing manipulations, whereas other facilities may not have such supplies and require more steps in the procedure and more safety precautions. Know what supplies are on hand and know how to use them.

Automated Devices

Automated devices used in TPN preparation can compound the base solutions, additives, or both. TPN compounders can be stand-alone automation, or they can be used in conjunction with compounding software. What follow are a few examples of different TPN compounders.

Automix 3+3

Clinitec has developed TPN software that can control the automated TPN Automix compounder. The Automix compounder is linked to a computer that controls how much is pumped into a TPN bag. First, the physician writes a TPN order that goes to the pharmacy. The pharmacist or certified pharmacy technician enters this information into the Clinitec computer, which then calculates how much of each ingredient is to be added. The computer displays warnings if any of the preprogrammed levels are off, including any precipitation problems. Then a label is printed out and checked by another pharmacist, or possibly two. The Automix is also available as a stand-alone compounder. In this case the technician manually inputs the volumes of the base solutions and the compounder pumps these volumes into the TPN bag.

After the labels are checked, the technician programs the Automix compounder for the correct patient, hangs the correct-size bag, and then pushes the Start button. The Automix compounder begins to push the fluid out of the base component bags into the TPN bag, which hangs on a hook that actually weighs the TPN bag as it is being pumped.

The compounder uses each base component's **specific gravity** to pump the correct amount into the TPN bag. For example, amino acids have a specific gravity of 1.07 mg/mL. If the total amount of amino acids needed in the TPN is 84 mL, we multiply $84 \times 1.07 = 89.88$ mg. After the Automix compounder measures that amount of amino acid, it automatically moves on to the next solution that needs to be pumped into the IV bag. As a safety feature, the Automix compounder also gives an alarm if a solution does not have the same specific gravity for which it is programmed. For example, if a bag of SWFI is hung (specific gravity 1.00) instead of a bag of dextrose 70% (specific gravity 1.24), then the machine would give an alarm to inform the user that the specific gravities do not match, which would indicate a medication error.

Other compounders similar to the Automix are B. Braun's Pinnacle compounder and Abbott's Nitrimix Macro.

Micromix

The Micromix compounder is for TPN additives and can add up to 10 different additives to the bag. This significantly reduces the number of syringes that must be drawn for each TPN. As long as the computer has been correctly programmed, the error rate is reduced. The Micromix compounder adds the additives to the TPN bag using the specific gravity of each additive. It works similarly to the Automix compounder, but with the greater accuracy needed for additives.

The Micromix compounder can pump as little as 2 mL correctly into a TPN bag and can measure to tenths (0.1 mL). The Micromix compounder is designed to add medications in the order programmed and to flush the lines between the different additives. Even though the Micromix compounder can add up to 10 additives, the IV technician usually still must pull a couple of additives in by hand.

Other compounders, such as BAXA's Exacta-Mix, compound and add both the base solution and additives to the TPN bag.

CONCLUSION

Certain patients in institutional settings must receive their daily nutrition from a TPN. These orders must be precise and can become quite complicated due to the sheer number of ingredients or additives involved. While some facilities now use automated technology to aid in the preparation of TPN orders, you must still be competent in this area if you will be using such equipment.

PROFILES OF PRACTICE

TPNs are considered an acute treatment, one with a specific length of duration, in most cases. Controversy has risen, however, as some physicians use TPNs to extend the life of a small number of children born with nonexistent or severely birth-deformed intestines. The oldest of these patients turned 8 years old in 2003.

CHAPTER TERMS

central line IV access directly through a central blood vessel
hyperglycemia a high level of glucose in the body
hypoglycemia a low level of glucose in the body
neonate a newborn baby

peripheral line IV access through peripheral veins in the arms, legs, hands, or feet
protocol the standard plan for a course of medical treatment
specific gravity the weight of a substance compared (as a ratio) with that of an equal volume of water

CHAPTER REVIEW QUESTIONS

MULTIPLE CHOICE

1. What does TPN stand for?
   a. total purchasable nutrition
   b. total parenteral naturalism
   c. total parenteral nutrition
   d. the parenteral nutrition
   e. total parental nutrition

2. What is not another name for TPN?
   a. the food bag
   b. total parenteral nutrition
   c. hyperalimentation bag
   d. hyperal
   e. bag

3. What two additives should never be mixed closely together?
   a. potassium chloride and potassium phosphate
   b. potassium chloride and calcium gluconate
   c. calcium gluconate and potassium chloride
   d. potassium phosphate and calcium gluconate
   e. calcium chloride and magnesium sulfate

4. In a hospital, who is responsible for writing a TPN?
   a. IV technicians
   b. pharmacists

   c. nurses
   d. physicians
   e. nurse practitioners

5. In a hospital, who is primarily responsible for compounding TPNs?
   a. IV technicians
   b. pharmacists
   c. nurses
   d. physicians
   e. pharmacy residents

6. Which of the following patients is a possible candidate for a TPN?
   a. a cancer patient
   b. a neonatal patient
   c. a surgical patient
   d. a pregnant patient
   e. all of the above

7. Which the following can cause precipitation when added to closely behind phosphate?
   a. sodium
   b. potassium
   c. calcium

d. multivitamin
e. trace elements

8. What additive should be added last to a TPN?

a. potassium chloride
b. potassium phosphates

c. calcium gluconate
(d.) multivitamin for injection
e. dextrose

MATCHING

Indicate whether each item is an additive (A) or a base (B) component. Put the appropriate letter by the additive or the base. Answers may be used more than once.

1. _____B_____ sterile water
2. _____A_____ sodium acetate
3. _____A_____ sodium chloride
4. _____A_____ sodium phosphate
5. _____B_____ TrophAmine 6%
6. _____A_____ potassium acetate
7. _____A_____ potassium chloride
8. _____B_____ dextrose 70%
9. _____A_____ potassium phosphate
10. _____A_____ magnesium sulfate
11. _____A_____ calcium gluconate
12. _____B_____ amino acids 10%

13. _____B_____ heparin
14. _____A_____ zinc
15. _____A_____ trace elements
16. _____A_____ chromium
17. _____B_____ lipids 20%
18. _____A_____ copper
19. _____A_____ multivitamin for injection
20. _____B_____ insulin
21. _____B_____ dextrose 50%
22. _____B_____ Pepcid

A. additive
B. base component

LABORATORY ACTIVITIES

1. What two electrolytes should not be mixed directly after the other when compounding a TPN? Why?

Potassium phosphate and calcium gluconase Because they are incompatibles can causes formation of insoluble salt.

2. TPN Order #1

Amino acids 8.5%	411.5 mL
Dextrose 50%	400.0 mL
Lipids 10%	250.0 mL
SWFI	305.6 mL
NaCl 4 mEq/mL	30 mEq 120 ml
Na phosphate 3 mM/mL	27 mM 81 ml
Ca gluconate 0.465 mEq/mL	4.65 mEq =2.162
Insulin, Regular 100 U/mL	35 units 0.35 ml
MVI-12	10 mL
Trace elements–5	1 mL

What is the total volume for this TPN order?

1581.61 ml

Compound this TPN order using proper sterile technique.

_____
_____
_____
_____

3. TPN Order #2

Amino acids 15%	562.6 mL
Dextrose 70%	456.9 mL
SWFI	267.8 mL
Na acetate 2 mEq/mL	14 mEq 28 ml
KCl 2 mEq/mL	10 mEq 20 ml
Magnesium sulfate 50% 4.06 mEq/mL	8.12 mEq 2 ml
Ca gluconate 0.465 mEq/mL	3.813 mEq 11.77
K phosphate 4.4 mEq/mL	8.8 mEq 2 ml
Trace elements–5	1 mL
MVI-12	10 mL

What is the total volume of this TPN order?

1352.07 ml

Compound this TPN order using proper sterile technique. *Aseptic Technique*

_____
_____
_____
_____

4. TPN Order #3

Amino acids 15%	1000 mL
Dextrose 70%	571.4 mL
Lipids 20%	250 mL
SWFI	105.6 mL
Ca gluconate 0.465 mEq/mL ✗	12 mEq 5.58 ml
Magnesium sulfate 50% 4.06 mEq/mL ✗	16 mEq 64.96
NaCl 4 mEq/mL ✗	80 mEq =320.0
Na phosphate 3 mM/mL ✗	20 mM =60.0
Na acetate 2 mEq/mL ✗	50 mEq 100
MVI-12	10 mL
Trace elements–5	1 mL
Insulin, Regular	38 units 0.38

What is the total volume of this TPN order?

_____ 2488.92 ml _____

(margin note: 10blank 1 ml)

Compound this TPN order using proper sterile technique. *Aseptic Technique*

_____
_____
_____
_____

5. TPN Order #4

Amino acids 15%	750 mL
Dextrose 70%	571.4 mL
Lipids 10%	250 mL
SWFI	234.8 mL
Ca gluconate 0.465 mEq/mL ✗	12 mEq 5.58
NaCl 4 mEq/mL ✗	20 mEq 80

K phosphate 4.4 mEq/mL	✗	27 mEq 118.80
Na acetate 2 mEq/mL	✗	32 mEq 64
MVI-12		10 mL
Trace elements–5		1 mL
Insulin, Regular	0.78	78 units 78÷100 0.78

What is the total volume of this TPN order?

_____ 2086.36 ml _____

Compound the above TPN order using proper sterile technique. *Aseptic Technique*

_____
_____
_____
_____

6. TPN Order #5

Amino acids 15%		500 mL
Dextrose 70%		571.4 mL
Lipids 10%		250 mL
SWFI		154.6 mL
Magnesium sulfate 50% 4.06 mEq/mL	✗	16 mEq 64.96
NaCl 4 mEq/mL	✗	60 mEq 240.0
Na phosphate 3 mM/mL		30 mM
Ca gluconate 0.465 mEq/mL	✗	12 mEq 5.58
Na acetate 2 mEq/mL	✗	10 mEq 20.0
MVI-12		10 mL
Trace elements–5		1 mL
Insulin, Regular	0.78	78 units

What is the total volume of this TPN order?

_____ 1848.32 ml _____

Compound this TPN order using proper sterile technique. *Aseptic Technique*

_____
_____
_____
_____

Chemotherapy

After completing this chapter, you should be able to:

- Describe what happens with cancer and cells.
- Explain how cytotoxic agents are used to treat cancer.
- Explain safety procedures for handling chemotherapy agents.
- Describe types of biological safety cabinets.
- Discuss appropriate procedures for preparing chemotherapy agents.
- List the hazards involved with preparing chemotherapy agents.
- Describe how to clean a chemotherapy spill.

Introduction

Cancer cells develop because of damage to DNA that causes cells in a part of the body to begin to grow out of control. Most cancers produce tumors, but some, such as leukemia, do not. Various types of cancer behave differently, grow at different rates, and respond to different treatments. This is why they require treatment that is specific to the cancer type. The earlier a cancer is found and treatment begins, the better are the chances for survival. The treatment for cancer is also difficult. There are many different types of cancer; the treatment may range from removing the **malignant** cells to **chemotherapy** and radiation.

INFORMATION

The National Pharmacy Technician Association offers an ACPE-accredited Chemo Certification course. For more information on becoming a chemo certified pharmacy technician, visit www.pharmacytechnician.org/chemo or call 1-888-247-8700.

The following is a partial list of types of cancer:

Bladder cancer	Lymphoma
Bone cancer	Melanoma
Brain cancer	Multiple myeloma
Breast cancer	Oral cancer
Cervical cancer	Ovarian cancer
Colon cancer	Pancreatic cancer
Esophageal cancer	Pharyngeal cancer
Extrahepatic bile duct cancer	Prostate cancer
Gallbladder cancer	Rectal cancer
Hodgkin's disease	Skin cancer
Kidney cancer	Stomach cancer
Laryngeal cancer	Testicular cancer
Leukemia	Uterine cancer
Liver cancer	Vaginal cancer
Lung cancer	Vulvar cancer

Several viruses are also known to be linked to cancer:

- Long-standing liver infection with the hepatitis virus can lead to cancer of the liver.
- A variety of the herpes virus, the Epstein-Barr virus, causes infectious mononucleosis and has been implicated in non-Hodgkin's lymphomas and nasopharyngeal cancer.
- The human immunodeficiency virus is associated with an increased risk of developing several cancers, especially Kaposi's sarcoma and non-Hodgkin's lymphoma.
- Human papilloma viruses have been linked to cancers of the cervix, vulva, and penis.

Although cancer is one of the primary reasons a patient will receive chemotherapy treatment, it is not the only reason. Chemotherapy may also be used to treat rheumatoid arthritis, lupus, psoriasis, and other autoimmune diseases. Our focus, however, will follow suit with aseptic preparation in the IV realm, which is typically used for patients with cancer.

The general idea of chemotherapy is to kill the tumor or the malignant cells without causing more damage than necessary to the patient's healthy cells. There is no cure for cancer, yet treatment with potent medications such as cytotoxic agents and antineoplastics can often suppress symptoms and provide better quality of life for the patient.

Some cancer types tend to affect a certain population more than others. For example, children tend to be the patients diagnosed with leukemia, while women get breast, ovarian, and uterine cancer; men are more at risk for prostate and colon cancer; and smokers have a higher incidence of lung cancer. Other cancers affect populations uniformly, such as brain tumors, liver cancer, and kidney cancer.

With a significant amount of the population being diagnosed with cancer, compounding **cytotoxic** agents is becoming a more common practice. This chapter is designed to help IV technicians protect themselves while also providing the best possible care for the patient.

Cytotoxic Agents

Cytotoxic agents, or **antineoplastics**, are used to treat patients with various forms of cancer. Chemotherapy drugs are extremely toxic to cells, and specific drugs are indicated for specific tumors or cells. The idea behind cytotoxic drugs is to kill the cancer or tumor without killing the patient. Unfortunately, chemotherapeutic agents cannot tell the difference between a healthy cell and a sick cell. This is why some patients succeed in eliminating the cancer but also have unwanted side effects such as hair loss.

Generally speaking, there are two classes of antineoplastic agents:

Cycle-Phase–Nonspecific Agents—These agents work on a cell at any time during the cell's cycle. There are five main types:
- Nitrogen mustards
- Ethylenimines
- Alkyl sulfonates
- Triazenes
- Nitrosoureas

Cycle-Phase–Specific Agents—These agents work on a cell during a specific cycle (most are nonresting). These agents are indicated for rapidly growing tumors where there is a high growth period. Antimetabolites are most commonly used for these types of tumors. Some examples are etoposide, hydroxyurea, vincristine, and vinblastine.

Take care when working with all antineoplastic agents, as they are potentially mutagenic (can cause cells to mutate), **carcinogenic** (can cause cancer), **teratogenic** (can cause birth defects), and immunosuppressive.

The following is a list of some common cytotoxic medications that the IV technician may come across:

Asparaginase (Elspar)
Bleomycin (Blenoxane)
Carboplatin (Paraplatin)
Carmustine (BiCNU)
Cisplatin (Platinol)
Cladribine (Leustatin)
Cyclophosphamide (Cytoxan, Neosar)
Dacarbazine (DTIC-Dome)
Dactinomycin (Actinomycin D)
Daunorubicin (Cerubidine)
Doxorubicin (Adriamycin, Doxil, Rubex, hydroxydaunomycin, hydroxydoxorubicin)
Estramustine (Estracyt)
Etoposide (VePesid, Etopophos)
Floxuridine (FUDR, fluorodeoxyuridine)
Fluorouracil (5FU)
Gemcitabine (Gemzar)
Idarubicin (Idamycin)
Ifosfamide (Ifex)
Mesna (Mesnex)
Methotrexate (MTX, Amethopterin)
Mitomycin (mitomycin-C, Mutamycin)
Paclitaxel (Taxol)
Plicamycin (Mithramycin)
Rituximab (Rituxan)
Thiotepa (Thioplex)
Vidarabine (Vira-A)
Vinblastine (Velban)
Vincristine (Vincasar, Oncovin)

Compounding Chemotherapy Medications

Compounding chemotherapy medications is a necessity for any technician preparing sterile products. When compounded properly and according to safety guidelines, chemotherapy preparation is no more dangerous to the preparer than the compounding of other sterile products. It is important to remember, however, that cytotoxic agents are toxic and are deadly to cells. The risks are great if these products come into contact with human skin. Mixing chemotherapeutic agents requires a strict degree of carefulness to avoid harm to the personnel preparing these products.

As with most medication orders, the physician initiates a chemotherapy drug order (Figure 8-1). The order is then sent to the pharmacy, where the pharmacist double-checks the order to ensure that it is written correctly. Then the IV technician begins to gather the necessary materials to compound the chemotherapy medication.

Preparation Areas

Facilities that compound chemotherapeutic agents are subjected to at least the same stringent requirements for the clean room atmosphere where the mixing of regular IVs takes place. There are necessary additions, however, such as biohazard waste containers, spill kits, special gloves, shower apparatus, dispensing pins, and other related supplies. Again, it is very important to become familiar with USP 797 guidelines and keep up to date with any revisions; these guidelines also apply to chemotherapeutic preparations.

Biological Safety Cabinets

Chemotherapy medications are compounded in a **biological safety cabinet (BSC)** (Figure 8-2) or vertical airflow hood. BSCs are designed to provide personnel, product, and environmental protection when proper procedures are followed. BSCs provide an ISO Class 5 environment.

A chemotherapy mat (**chemo mat**) is placed inside the BSC to absorb any leaks or spills. The same sterile materials used in the IV hood may also be used in the BSC.

There are several types of biological safety cabinets. BSCs are available in Class I, II, or III. Table 8-1 lists the differences according to risk assessment. Chemotherapy agents should be prepared in a class II BSC, which is a vertical airflow cabinet containing high-efficiency particulate air (HEPA) filters.

The main difference among BSCs is that some are vented directly to the outside and others filter the air again before circulating it back into the clean room air. This type of hood has a front glass cover (view screen) that is brought down when mixing to leave a 6-in. opening through which to enter and work.

- The *Class I BSC* provides personnel and environmental protection but no product protection. It is similar in air movement to a chemical fume hood but has a HEPA filter in the exhaust system to protect the environment.
- The *Class II BSC* provides personnel, environmental, and product protection. Airflow is drawn from around the operator into the front grille of the cabinet, which provides personnel protection. In addition, the downward laminar flow of HEPA-filtered air provides product protection by minimizing the chance of cross-contamination along the work surface of the cabinet.
- The *Class III BSC* was designed for work with biosafety level 4 microbiological agents and provides maximum protection to the environment and the worker. It is a gas-tight enclosure with a nonopening view window.

These BSCs work great depending on how many and what types of chemotherapy agents are being compounded in the clean room. For institutions that do not

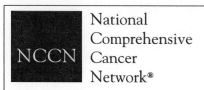

Chemotherapy Order Template™
Breast Cancer
AC (DOXOrubicin/Cyclophosphamide) Every 21 Days
→DOCEtaxel Every 21 Days + Trastuzumab

AC (DOXOrubicin/Cyclophosphamide) Every 21 Days Course
page 1 of 2

INDICATION:	REFERENCES:	NCCN SUPPORTIVE CARE:
Adjuvant	1. <u>NCCN Clinical Practice Guidelines in Oncology™ Breast Cancer. V.1.2009.</u> 2. <u>Robert N, et al. *J Clin Oncol.* 2007; 25(18S):19647.</u>[b]	1. *Emetic Risk:* Day 1 High 2. *Fever Neutropenia Risk:* Intermediate

CHEMOTHERAPY REGIMEN
21-day cycle for 4 cycles

- **DOXOrubicin** 60 mg/m^2 IV Push on Day 1
- See *Safety Parameters and Special Instructions* for information on slow IV Push administration.
- **Cyclophosphamide** 600 mg/m^2 IV over 30 minutes on Day 1
- Oral hydration is strongly encouraged with cyclophosphamide; poorly hydrated patients may need supplemental IV hydration. Patients should attain combined oral and IV hydration of 2 – 3 L/day on day of chemotherapy. See *Other Supportive Therapy* for example of recommended hydration.

This course is 4 cycles of AC (DOXOrubicin and cyclophosphamide) Every 21 Days.
DOCEtaxel Every 21 Days and trastuzumab course is initiated following completion of this course.
Please see Order Template BRS27b for DOCEtaxel Every 21 Days and trastuzumab course.

SUPPORTIVE CARE

Antiemetic therapy (See www.nccn.org/professionals/physician_gls/PDF/antiemesis.pdf)

Days 1 – 4

- Aprepitant 125 mg PO or fosaprepitant 115 mg IV Day 1, aprepitant 80 mg PO Days 2 – 3
  AND
- Dexamethasone 12 mg PO/IV Days 1 –4
  AND
- 5-HT3 antagonist (recommended on days of highly emetogenic chemotherapy administration):
  Palonosetron 0.25 mg IV Day 1
  OR
  Dolasetron 100 mg PO or 1.8 mg/kg IV or 100 mg IV Day 1
  OR
  Granisetron 2 mg PO daily or 1 mg PO BID or 0.01 mg/kg (maximum 1 mg) IV daily Day 1 or transdermal patch containing 34.3 mg granisetron applied 24 – 48 hours prior to first dose of chemotherapy (patch supplies 5 days of therapeutic drug starting 24 hours after application)
  OR
  Ondansetron 16 – 24 mg PO or 8 – 12 mg (maximum 32 mg/day) IV Day 1
  AND
- ± Lorazepam 0.5 – 2 mg PO/IV or sublingual every 4 or every 6 hours as needed Days 1 – 4
  AND
- ± H$_2$ blocker or proton pump inhibitor

Template continued on page 2

FIGURE 8-1 Chemotherapy order

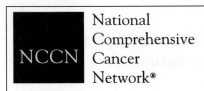

Chemotherapy Order Template™
Breast Cancer
AC (DOXOrubicin/Cyclophosphamide) Every 21 Days
→DOCEtaxel Every 21 Days + Trastuzumab

BRS27a

AC (DOXOrubicin/Cyclophosphamide) Every 21 Days Course
page 2 of 2

PRN for breakthrough: Patients should be given at least one medication in a different category than that given above to have as needed for breakthrough. Please consult the NCCN Clinical Practice Guidelines in Oncology™ Antiemesis for appropriate antiemetic therapy.

Myeloid growth factor therapy (See www.nccn.org/professionals/physician_gls/PDF/myeloid_growth.pdf)

CSFs not generally recommended as primary prophylaxis based on FN risk of chemotherapy regimen. For more information on prophylaxis of FN, refer to NCCN Clinical Practice Guidelines in Oncology™ Myeloid Growth Factors and Appendix C to the NCCN Chemotherapy Order Templates.

Other Supportive Therapy

- F or cyclophosphamide: *Example of recommended hydration*: Sodium chloride 0.9% infused IV at a rate of 1.5 – 3 mL/kg/hour for a total of 500 mL on day of chemotherapy.

MONITORING AND HOLD PARAMETERS

- CBC with differential should be assessed routinely for potential dose evaluation.
- For DOXOrubicin:
  o DOXOrubicin is an anthracycline. Cumulative anthracycline dosage should be monitored.
  o Ejection fraction should be assessed prior to initiation of treatment and as clinically indicated.
  o Liver function should be assessed prior to each cycle for potential dose evaluation.
- For cyclophosphamide: Renal function should be assessed prior to each cycle for potential dose evaluation.

SAFETY PARAMETERS AND SPECIAL INSTRUCTIONS

- F or DOXOrubicin:
  o **DOXOrubicin is a vesicant.**
  o This agent is administered IV Push. The preferred IV Push method for a vesicant is administration through the side port of a freely flowing IV; alternatively, the drug can be administered via direct IV push.
- For aprepitant and fosaprepitant: Refer to Appendix D for specific information regarding associated drug interactions.

FIGURE 8-1 Chemotherapy order (*continued*)

compound cytotoxic agents on a regular basis, a BSC that recirculates the filtered air back into the room will suffice. However, if 10 or more cytotoxic agents are being compounded weekly, then a BSC that vents directly to the outside is preferred.

BSCs must be validated or certified for integrity at least every 6 months or if the hood is moved, since relocating a BSC may break the HEPA filter seals or otherwise damage the filters or the cabinet.

BSCs blow clean air from the top of the hood vertically toward the bottom of the hood, unlike the laminar airflow hood, which blows clean air horizontally toward the IV technician. With this vertical flow of air, the cytotoxic fumes are kept in the hood. The IV technician must always keep the direction of the airflow in mind to prevent **shadowing**. Shadowing occurs when airflow in the BSC is blocked.

A *compounding aseptic containment isolator* or CACI is a specially designed airflow hood that helps restrict free movement of contaminants. It is a contained unit in which the operator slips his or her hands into long, glovelike parts whose surface is completely encompassed inside the hood. This type of hood is highly favored by USP 797 guidelines as appropriate for use in multitasking situations. CACI's requires less space, have monitoring controls, and are basically self-contained.

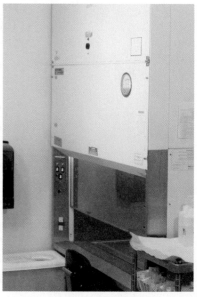

FIGURE 8-2 Biological safety cabinet

Table 8–1   Comparison of Biological Safety Cabinet Characteristics

BIOLOGICAL SAFETY CABINET CLASS	FACE VELOCITY (ft/min)	AIRFLOW PATTERN	NONVOLATILE TOXIC CHEMICALS AND RADIONUCLIDES	APPLICATION TO VOLATILE TOXIC CHEMICALS AND RADIONUCLIDES
I	75	In at the front; exhausted through HEPA to the outside or into the room through HEPA	Yes	Yes
II, A	75	Seventy percent recirculated to the cabinet work area through HEPA; the 30% balance can be through HEPA back into the room or to the outside through a thimble unit	Yes	No
II, B1	100	Exhaust cabinet air must pass through a dedicated duct to the outside through a HEPA filter	Yes	Yes (minute amounts)
II, B2	100	No recirculation; total exhaust to the outside through the hard duct and a HEPA filter	Yes	Yes (small amounts)
II, B3	100	Same as II, A, but plenums are under negative pressure to the room; exhaust air is thimble-ducted to the outside through a HEPA filter	Yes	Yes (minute amounts)
III	N/A	Supply air inlets and hard duct are exhausted to the outside through two HEPA filters in series	Yes	Yes (small amounts)

Proper Use of the Biological Safety Cabinet

The BSC requires the same consideration as the LAH while in operation. Some key points to keep in mind are as follows:

- Keep the insides and tops of BSCs free of unnecessary equipment or supplies.
- Turn off all ultraviolet lights whenever the laboratory is occupied.
- Wash hands and arms with germicidal soap before and after work in the BSC.
- Wear a long-sleeved gown with tight-fitting cuffs and sterile gloves as part of your PPE.
- Do not eat, drink, apply cosmetics or lip balm, store food, or smoke in the laboratory.
- Dispose of sharps in a puncture-resistant chemotherapy container. Do not resheath or remove used needles; insert the whole assembly into the container.
- Clean up spills immediately.
- Properly dispose of all waste materials into biohazard containers.
- Disinfect interior surfaces of the work area using sterile water and 70% isopropyl alcohol or another appropriate disinfectant.
- Place everything you need for the complete procedure in the cabinet before starting work and limit passing in or out through the air barrier until the procedure is completed.
- Set the view screen at the proper height.
- Wait 5 minutes after you have placed all materials in the BSC before beginning work. This will enable the BSC to purge airborne contaminants from the work area.
- Work as far to the back of the BSC workspace as possible.
- Do not work in a BSC while a warning light or alarm is signaling.
- After you complete your work, enclose or cover all equipment and materials. Allow the BSC to run for 5 minutes to purge airborne contaminants from the work area.
- Periodically decontaminate under work grills and work surfaces if these parts are removable.
- When the blower is shut off, the air barrier is destroyed. Within seconds, the inside of the cabinet becomes contaminated with microorganisms from the laboratory. For this reason, the BSC is generally operated with the blower turned on 24 hours a day.

Preparing to Use the Hood

1. Turn off ultraviolet light as soon as you enter the room.
2. Check the flow alarm system audio and visual alarm function (if the unit is so equipped).
3. Decontaminate readily accessible interior surfaces with a disinfectant appropriate for the agents or suspected agents present and wait at least 10 minutes.

As you are now aware, frequent cleaning is paramount in clean room settings. The following is a basic procedure you can use. Facilities may have slight variations, but the basic procedure is universally acceptable.

Cleaning and Decontaminating the Biological Safety Cabinet (Figure 8-3)

1. Dress for cytotoxic drug preparation using hair cover, mask, shoe covers, and a chemotherapy-specific gown.
2. Wash your hands thoroughly with a germicidal cleanser, dry properly, then apply chemotherapy gloves and the appropriate sterile gloves.

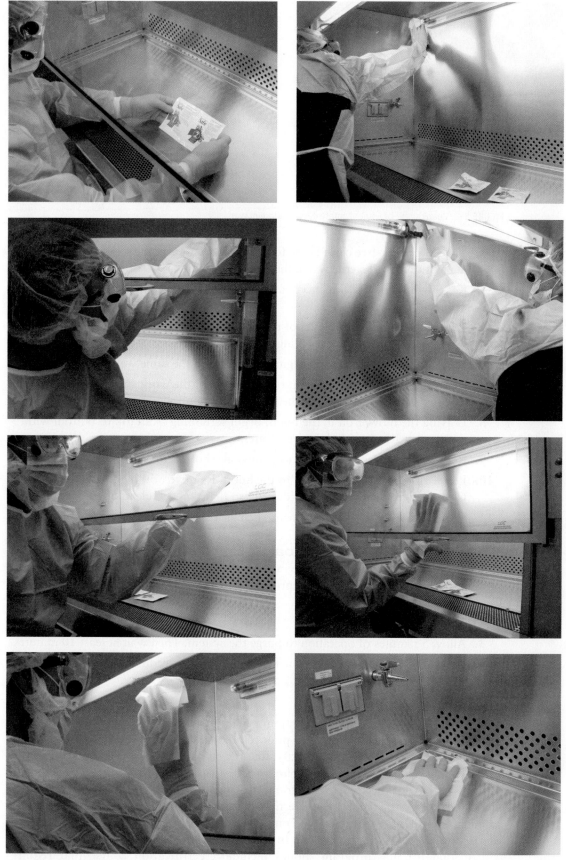

FIGURE 8-3 Cleaning the biological safety cabinet

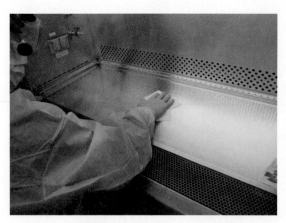 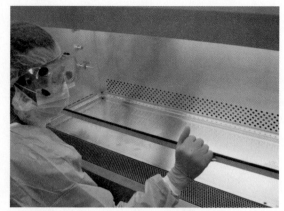

FIGURE 8-3 Cleaning the biological safety cabinet (*continued*)

3. Use a clean, lint-free cloth in the following steps. Repeat the following steps twice, the first time with sterile water, the second time with 70% isopropyl alcohol.

4. Keeping in mind the direction of the airflow, begin cleaning the bar at the top of the hood.

5. Then move to the back panel of the hood. Begin cleaning at the top of the panel in a side-to-side motion, working toward the bottom.

6. Move to the side panels and begin cleaning them the same way as the back panel.

7. Clean the work surface area. Start at the back of the work surface area, cleaning side to side, working toward the front of the hood.

8. Leaving the blower on in the hood, begin scrubbing from top to bottom with the cleaner. Rinse with deionized water.

9. Repeat this process with 70% isopropyl alcohol.

10. Leave all movable parts inside of the hood. Remove nothing from the hood. Clean and move items to the side only so that you can clean other parts.

11. Clean heavily contaminated areas, such as a spillage trough, twice.

Shutting Down the Biological Safety Cabinet

1. Decontaminate all items in the interior work area and readily accessible interior surfaces with a disinfectant appropriate for the agents or suspected agents present, then remove them.

2. Turn on the ultraviolet light.

3. Allow 5 minutes of operation to purge the system. Then wait at least 10 minutes.

4. Turn off the BSC blower if your facility has this procedure.

Personnel Training

It is extremely important to properly train personnel who will be mixing chemotherapy products and assess their competency prior to mixing. Competency should be assessed at least annually or any time it is suspected that the employee is not following proper protocol. Highly skilled and trained employees are essential for safety in the chemotherapy process. As part of the training program, it is highly recommended to review and test employees for competency to ensure that they have been adequately trained. Proper training, competency assessment, and ongoing education regarding chemotherapy preparation cannot be emphasized enough for the pharmacy technician working in this area.

A good training program should include a certification course that requires recertification on a regular basis, such as yearly. The trainer of such programs should, at a minimum, have several years of experience and be quite knowledgeable with chemotherapy drugs as well as with other related information regarding chemotherapy preparation.

Chemotherapy preparation is an ongoing, complex process with changes occurring constantly. This field also requires knowledge of related information such as chemotherapy procurement, storage, safe handling procedures, and preparation and waste guidelines for chemotherapy procedures. Up-to-date information relating to chemotherapy preparation, policies, procedures, regulations, drugs, and other topics should be accessible to personnel at all times and maintained by the workplace.

Attire

Unlike other types of sterile products, compounding chemotherapy drugs requires specific attire (Figure 8-4). In addition to the sterile cap and shoe covers, the IV technician must also wear a lint-free gown, goggles, and gloves. The additional gowning attire is designed to protect the IV technician in a worst-case scenario. Many chemotherapy drugs are irritants; acute side effects from skin exposure include skin irritation, blistering, and discoloration.

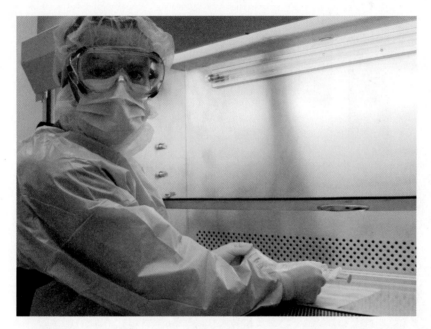

FIGURE 8-4 Chemotherapy attire

The following are some guidelines for chemotherapy attire:

- When gowning up for a chemotherapy preparation, use a low-permeability, solid-front gown that ties in the back.
- Wear disposable, high-cuff, latex chemotherapy or nitrile gloves when working with biohazards (latex gloves are permeable to organic solvents).
- Use the thickest gloves allowed by your workplace to protect against cuts and scratches without compromising dexterity.
- Wear two pairs of thinner gloves to permit safe removal of the outer pair in case of inadvertent contamination.
- Wear a disposable lab coat, closed and with the sleeves tucked into the gloves, while in the lab.
- Do not wear lab coats outside the laboratory.
- Wear eye protection, such as goggles provided by your workplace.

Workplace Wisdom

When you have brought materials into the BSC, do not bring them out again. You can leave them in the BSC until you use them, or dispose of them in the **yellow hazardous disposal container**. Do not put them back into the regular stock.

Withdrawing a Cytotoxic Agent

You must perform this procedure using proper aseptic technique (Figure 8-5):

1. Gather all materials needed for the manipulation.
2. Most important, remember the direction of the airflow. In the BSC the air flows downward. In order to manipulate items aseptically, you must not block the airflow. In other words, do not place your hands or fingers between items that must remain sterile and the direction of the airflow.
3. Swab the rubber top with alcohol. Allow the alcohol to dry.
4. Ensure that the needle is firmly attached to a Luer-lock syringe. Only Luer-lock syringes can be used to prepare chemotherapy.
5. Pull the plunger back on the syringe to approximately half the amount of drug needed.

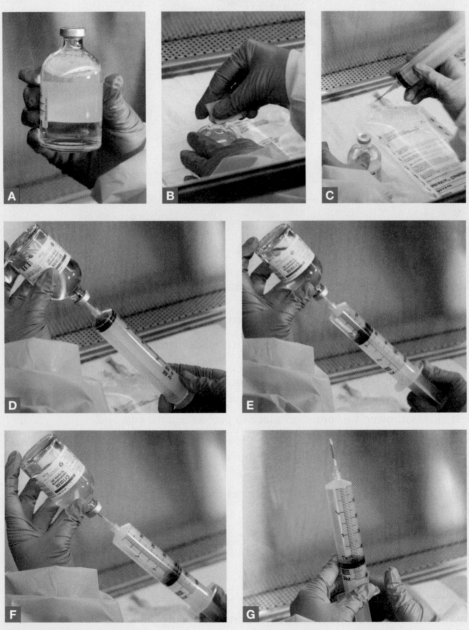

FIGURE 8-5 Withdrawing a cytotoxic agent

6. Never put a volume of air into the vial that is greater than or equal to the desired amount of cytotoxic agent that you need to withdraw. This will cause positive pressure in the bottle, creating **aerosolization** of the cytotoxic agent.

7. Remove the cap from the needle. Find the center of the stopper and insert the needle, bevel end up.

8. Turn the vial on its side so that clean air can blow directly on the sterile parts of the syringe and stopper.

9. Holding the syringe on the bottom side so as not to disrupt airflow, slowly add the air from the syringe into the vial. In some cases, it may be necessary to add the air 1 mL at a time.

10. Remove the desired amount of cytotoxic agent by pulling back on the plunger.

11. When the desired amount is reached, remove the needle from the vial.

12. Remove any air bubbles, using an empty evacuated container.

13. Recap the syringe.

14. Perform a final check.

Procedures for Handling Sterile Injectable Hazardous Drugs

Adhering to the following guidelines will help ensure that the chemotherapy is prepared properly with minimal chance of error or contamination to the product or the preparer.

- Ensure that syringes and IV sets have Luer-to-Luer connections (Figure 8-6).

- Do not fill syringes more than three-fourths full to prevent accidental separation of the plunger (Figure 8-7).

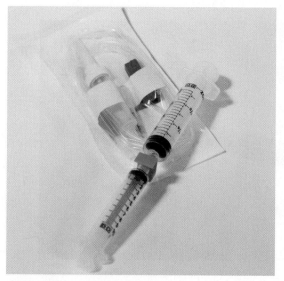

FIGURE 8-6 Luer-to-Luer syringe and intravenous set

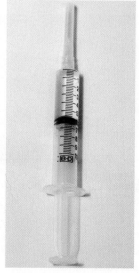

FIGURE 8-7 Properly filled syringe

- Use venting devices with 0.2-micron hydrophobic filters and 5-micron filter needles/straws for additional protection (Figure 8-8).

- Do not use ordinary vented needles.

- Dispense final products in a ready-to-administer form.

- Wipe the outsides of containers and IV sets with moist gauze (70% alcohol) to remove any inadvertent contamination. Also wipe all IV ports clean and cover them with a foil cap (Figure 8-9).

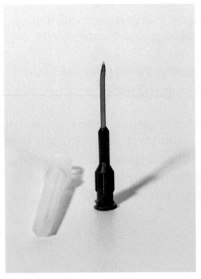

FIGURE 8-8 Venting devices

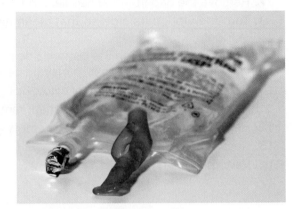

FIGURE 8-9 Covered intravenous ports

- Label final products, place them in a sealable zip-lock container, and label them as hazardous drugs.
- Do not use IV containers designed with venting tubes, to prevent possible spillage.
- Perform work with hazardous drugs in a BSC on a disposable, plastic-backed paper liner, which you should change after a spill or when sterile compounding is complete (Figure 8-10).
- Attach and prime any IV tubing BEFORE adding chemotherapy drug to the solution or container.

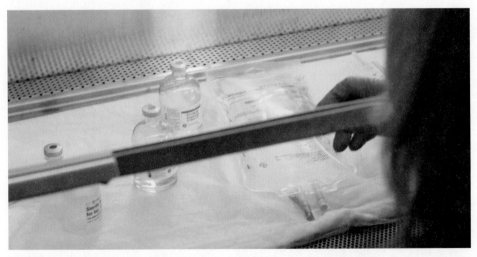

FIGURE 8-10 Final product

PhaSeal

Many pharmacy workplaces use a device known as the PhaSeal (Figures 8-11, 8-12, and 8-13). This closed-system transfer device, distributed by Carmel Pharma, Inc., is designed to reduce or eliminate human exposure to hazardous drugs. Currently, PhaSeal is the only device with clinical evidence proven to meet NIOSH's definition of a closed-system transfer device. The PhaSeal is a set of disposable containment devices used in drug mixing and administration that connect the original drug vial, the syringe, and the IV injection or infusion set together in a sealed pathway. It is constructed with a double membrane that prevents drug leakage; an expansion chamber equalizes the pressure in the system to prevent aerosols.

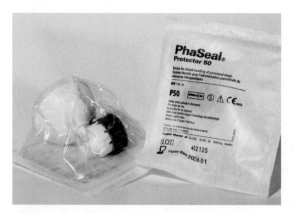

FIGURE 8-11 PhaSeal Protector 50 protected needle for sealed transfer of fluids from vial to syringe and syringe to delivery device; Luer-lock connector.

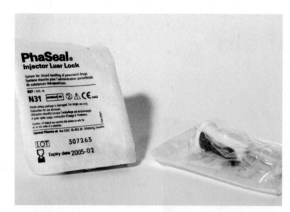

FIGURE 8-12 PhaSeal Injector Luer-lock expansion chamber for standard-neck vials and 50-mL syringes or smaller; holds up to 60 cc of air.

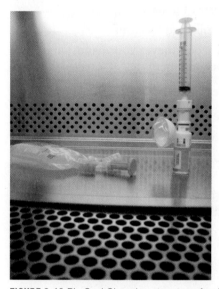

FIGURE 8-13 PhaSeal Closed-system transfer device

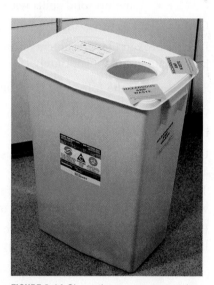

FIGURE 8-14 Chemotherapy waste container

Disposal of Cytotoxic Medications

Dispose of all cytotoxic medications and related supplies in a yellow, puncture-resistant hazardous container identified as a chemotherapy waste container (Figure 8-14). There are no exceptions. Chemotherapy waste includes the following:

- Discarded gloves
- Disposable gowns
- Disposable goggles
- Any other disposable material used during chemotherapy preparation or administration, such as IV bags/bottles, tubing, needles, syringes, and any unbreakable items

Place all cytotoxic waste items in a sealed zip-lock bag before putting them in the hazardous waste container. Dispose of needles and syringes in a hazardous puncture-proof sharps container without clipping or capping them.

Chemotherapy Spills

The Occupational Safety and Health Administration (OSHA) recommends that chemotherapy spill kits (Figure 8-15) be kept available at all times in areas in which cytotoxic compounding or administration occurs. The spill kit must be clearly labeled and contain the following items:

- Chemical splash goggles
- Low-**permeability** disposable gown and shoe covers or coveralls

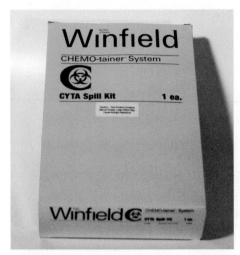

FIGURE 8-15 Chemotherapy spill kit

- Two pairs of gloves (utility and latex gloves)
- Two sheets of absorbent, plastic-backed material
- 250-mL and 1-L spill control pillows
- Puncture-resistant sharps container
- Small scoop to collect glass fragments
- Two large, labeled, sealable hazardous drug waste disposal bags
- Appropriate respirator

There are two types of spills—large and small. The American Society of Health-System Pharmacists (ASHP) defines small spills as less than 5 mL or 5 g. Large spills are anything over 5 mL or 5 g.

OSHA suggests the following guidelines for cleaning small spills:

- Wipe up liquid spills with absorbent gauze pads.
- Wipe up solid spills with wet absorbent gauze.
- Clean spill areas three times using a detergent followed by clean water.
- Pick up broken glass fragments using a small scoop (never your hands) and place them in an appropriately labeled sharps container.

OSHA suggests the following guidelines for cleaning large spills:

- Gently cover liquid spills with absorbent sheets or spill-control pads or pillows.
- Clean up powder spills with damp cloths or towels.
- Use protective apparel, including respirators, if there is any suspicion of any airborne powder or aerosols.
- Thoroughly clean all contaminated surfaces three times with detergent and water. Avoid chemical inactivation in this setting.
- Place all contaminated absorbent sheets and other material in an appropriately labeled hazardous drug disposal bag.

ASHP Guidelines for Safe Handling of Cytotoxic Drugs

The ASHP *Technical Assistance Bulletin on Handling Cytotoxic and Hazardous Drugs* contains pertinent, valuable information. It is strongly advised that you become familiar with its content. This document provides several guidelines/suggestions from ASHP to help protect personnel and patients from accidental exposure, such as the following:

- Limit access.
- Identify and label all hazardous drugs.
- Educate the patient and family about any and all special precautions that might need to be taken.
- Have a written procedure in place for any chemotherapy spills along with a chemotherapy spill kit.
- Design facilities to prevent easy spillage and breakage (e.g., place chemotherapy drugs in a bin on a shelf rather than just on a shelf).
- Use a method for transportation designed to reduce spills, such as a cart with a rim.
- Maintain written policies and procedures for the preparation of chemotherapeutic agents.
- Conduct orientations for all employees to inform them about hazardous drugs.
- Implement yearly process validations to test the performance of the staff.

- Keep Material Safety Data Sheets (MSDS) for each individual hazardous drug easily accessible in the pharmacy.
- Engineer appropriate airflow and venting to protect the sterility of the product as well as to protect personnel from possible exposure.
- Require employees to wear appropriate apparel, including the following:
  - Gloves—disposable, sterile surgical latex, and powder free. ASHP recommends double-gloving (wearing two pairs of gloves).
  - Gown—disposable, lint-free, low-permeability fabric, with a solid front, long sleeves, and tight-fitting cuffs.
  - Respirator—must be worn if not working in a BSC.
  - Goggles—should be worn in situations in which personnel may be exposed to potential eye contact.
- Design policies to outline proper aseptic technique.
- Train personnel in procedures for preparing and dispensing noninjectable hazardous drugs.
- Train personnel in procedures in case of accidental skin or eye exposure to hazardous drugs.
- Ensure that all hazardous drugs bear a CAUTION label.

A Final Caution

If you are pregnant, nursing, or thinking about becoming pregnant, avoid compounding cytotoxic agents—both IV and oral. Many hospitals have set guidelines for employees that fit into these categories. Remember that most cytotoxic (antineoplastic) drugs target fast-growing cells, including the ovaries and sperm. In addition, some chemotherapy drugs are mutagenic, which may increase the risk of miscarriages and birth defects.

The following are other risks associated with the handling of chemotherapy drugs:

- The drug may get out of the container and into the air.
- The drug may enter the handler's body through inhalation, absorption, ingestion, or accidental injection.
- The drug may cause cell damage.

Pharmacy technicians can never be too careful when it comes to the safety and handling of chemotherapy drugs. Knowledge and practice are key.

CONCLUSION

Proper aseptic technique is necessary to protect both the patient and the preparer when compounding cytotoxic or antineoplastic agents used in chemotherapy. These drugs are designed with one primary purpose: to kill or damage cells; they are nondiscriminatory, in that they will damage the technician's cells just as easily as the targeted cells of the patient, if contact occurs. You must take special precautions when working with these agents; only experienced, trained, and validated technicians should be involved in the preparation of these products.

CHAPTER TERMS

aerosolization a process resulting in a suspension of small particles (liquid or powder) in the air

antineoplastic a drug intended to inhibit or prevent the maturation and proliferation of neoplasms that may become malignant

biological safety cabinet (BSC) a type of airflow hood in which chemotherapy drugs are compounded

carcinogenic producing a malignant new growth that arises from the epithelium, which is found in skin or, more commonly, the lining of body organs

chemo mat an absorbent mat used in the BSC over which the IV tech should compound cytotoxic agents so any spills can be absorbed

chemotherapy treatment of cancer with drugs (chemicals)

cytotoxic describes chemicals that are directly toxic to cells, preventing their reproduction or growth
malignant tending to become progressively worse and to result in death
permeability the property or state of being penetrable

shadowing the act of blocking airflow in the BSC
teratogenic tending to produce anomalies of formation
yellow hazardous disposal containers containers used to dispose of hazardous medications and the equipment used to compound them; these containers require special disposal

CHAPTER REVIEW QUESTIONS

MULTIPLE CHOICE

1. What types of patients are diagnosed with cancer?
   a. children
   b. women
   c. men
   d. geriatrics
   e. all of the above

2. What cells do chemotherapy agents target?
   a. all cells
   b. slow-growing cells
   c. fast-growing cells
   d. carcinoma cells
   e. plasma cells

3. Any syringe used in the preparation of cytotoxic drugs should not filled more than _____ full with chemotherapy drug.
   a. 1/4
   b. 1/2
   c. 2/3
   d. 3/4

4. When working in a biological safety cabinet (BSC), the IV technician must keep in mind the direction of the airflow to prevent shadowing. Where does shadowing occur in the BSC?
   a. from the front of the hood
   b. from the back of the hood
   c. from the top of the hood
   d. from behind the operator
   e. shadowing does not occur in a BSC

5. All chemotherapy drugs and waste must be disposed of in a _____.
   a. yellow hazardous disposal container
   b. red biohazard container
   c. blue recycle bin
   d. oversized medical waste container
   e. stainless steel cart

6. Needles and syringes used in the preparation of chemotherapy drugs should always be capped before being disposed of into a hazardous sharps container.
   a. true
   b. false

7. Who is responsible for writing a chemotherapy order?
   a. IV technician
   b. pharmacist
   c. nurse
   d. physician
   e. patient

8. Who is responsible for performing a final check on a chemotherapy medication?
   a. IV technician
   b. pharmacist
   c. nurse
   d. physician
   e. patient

9. The HEPA filter must be recertified every _____ or if the hood is moved.
   a. 2 years
   b. evening
   c. 6 months
   d. year
   e. other day

10. Final products should be labeled and placed in _____.
    a. a sealable zip-lock container
    b. an airtight glass container
    c. an opaque container to protect from light
    d. a container with a carry handle
    e. a stainless steel container

11. A large spill is considered anything over _____.
    a. 1 oz
    b. 10 mL
    c. 4 mL
    d. 5 mL

12. IV tubing should be attached to the IV bag after adding the chemotherapy drug.
    a. true
    b. false

13. A BSC provides the preparer an _____ air environment.
    a. ISO 3
    b. ISO 4
    c. ISO 5
    d. ISO 6

MATCHING

Match the following chemotherapy trade and generic drug names.

1. Bleomycin _e_
2. Carboplatin _l_
3. Carmustine _d_
4. Cisplatin _m_
5. Cyclophosphamide _g_
6. Dacarbazine _h_
7. Dactinomycin _b_
8. Daunorubicin _f_
9. Doxorubicin _c_
10. Etoposide _q_
11. Fluorouracil _a_
12. Ifosfamide _i_
13. Mesna _x_
14. Paclitaxel _o_
15. Rituximab _n_
16. Vinblastine _p_
17. Vincristine _k_

a. 5FU
b. Actinomycin
c. Adriamycin
d. BiCNU
e. Blenoxane
f. Cerubidine
g. Cytoxan
h. DTIC-Dome
i. Ifex
j. Mesnex
k. Oncovin
l. Paraplatin
m. Platinol
n. Rituxan
o. Taxol
p. Velban
q. VePesid

LABORATORY ACTIVITIES

1. Practice gowning and ungowning the proper PPE for preparing chemotherapy medications.

2. What size syringe (1, 3, 5, 10, 20, 30, 60 mL) would be used to draw up the following chemotherapy doses?

3. Using proper sterile technique for preparing hazardous drugs, compound the following orders:
   a. Hazardous powder 10 mg in D5W 50 mL
   b. Hazardous liquid 500 mg in NS 100 mL

	CHEMOTHERAPY DRUG VOLUME (mL)	SYRINGE NEEDED
a.	7.5	
b.	8.6	
c.	3.5	
d.	26.4	
e.	19.6	
f.	1.5	
g.	30	
h.	2.7	
i.	9.6	
j.	15	

4. Using proper sterile technique for preparing hazardous drugs, compound the following orders:
   a. Hazardous powder 7.5 mg in D5W 100 mL
   b. Hazardous powder 2 mg in NS 100 mL
   c. Hazardous liquid 200 mg in NS 100 mL
   d. Hazardous liquid 450 mg in D5W 100 mL
   e. Hazardous Powder 5.6 mg in D5W 50 mL
   f. Hazardous Powder 15 mg in NS 250 mL
   g. Hazardous liquid 700 mg in D5W 250 mL
   h. Hazardous liquid 932 mg in NS 1000 mL
   i. Hazardous Powder 0.0086 g in NS 250 mL
   j. Hazardous liquid 0.875 g in D5W 500 mL

5. A doctor orders etoposide 75 mg/m^2 per day for 5 days. The patient's body surface area is 1.2 m^2. Etoposide is available in a 20-mg/mL injection. How many milligrams have been ordered by the doctor, and how many milliliters would be drawn up by the technician to prepare the first dose?

_____

_____

_____

_____

_____

Quality Control and Assurance

After completing this chapter, you should be able to:

- Explain the necessity of quality control.
- State tasks that require quality assurance procedures.
- Describe how the pharmacy technician helps the pharmacist ensure the quality of all pharmaceutical services.
- List the principles of quality assurance to all pharmacy activities.
- List and explain the USP 797 risk levels for compounded sterile products.
- Compare the various ASHP risk levels for different compounded sterile preparations and the quality assurance requirements of each.

Introduction

Successful management of quality is not just the responsibility of the quality manager or the quality assurance department. Each and every person involved in the pharmacy must understand the inherent responsibility that accompanies pharmaceuticals and their production. Quality assurance activities are an absolute necessity in pharmacy. Each aspect of pharmacy requires quality measurements to ensure integrity of the process and the final product. As someone who is involved in compounding sterile products, you must be completely aware of the potential consequences of poor quality control. Although very important, practicing proper aseptic sterile technique is only one area subjected to quality control measures.

Crucial to any product that is manufactured and delivered to a patient population, including sterile compounds, is a set of testing activities that determines the integrity of both the production process and the quality of the final product. Through careful design and validation of both the process and process controls, a manufacturer can establish a high degree of confidence that all manufactured units from successive lots will be acceptable. Pharmacy is a highly regulated arena. Sterile product preparation, if conducted poorly, has the potential for producing contaminated products that can harm patients and personnel. Problems due to cross-contamination, such as infection and even death, can result if strict procedures that limit the possibility of such exposure are not followed.

The importance of approved quality control activities and measures cannot be emphasized enough in this text. Quality assurance should never be underestimated, nor should any part of the process skipped for any reason. To do so would compromise public and patient safety.

INFORMATION

Guidelines are constantly evolving and being adjusted by the various agencies. It is important to always review the current official guidelines, policies, and recommendations from each agency.

Elements of Quality in Pharmacy

All pharmacy personnel must understand the basic rules of pharmacy when it comes to medication error prevention.

The Seven Rights

The seven rights make up a simple checklist to be used at any point in the medication process. Ensuring that each item is correct allows very little room for error. The seven rights are as follows:

- Right patient
- Right medication
- Right dose
- Right route of administration
- Right time
- Right technique
- Right documentation

Know each one of these rights and do not forget them throughout your pharmacy career. Related criteria to the seven rights are considerations such as the correct therapy for the patient's condition (right reason) and stringent rules for compounding of medications (right technique).

Quality Assurance Functions

Numerous activities must be performed in order to ensure the integrity of the product and the production. These include written policies and procedures, documentation, personnel training, system checks, **process validation**, and daily assessment of all operations.

Quality Improvement

In each facility subjected to quality control measures, a process of quality improvement must also be in place. Quality improvement ensures that while processes are performed over time, integrity is not lost due to problems such as lack of training, equipment failure, outdated facilities, and other noncompliance issues. Essential to this process are activities such as monitoring trends, conducting audits, identifying and analyzing problems, taking corrective measures, conducting tests, and suggesting change. One area that has received a great deal of attention is medication errors, which are usually the result of a system failure. Many facilities constantly revise their processes in an effort to minimize errors by closely evaluating each and every step involved. This is just one example of where quality control measures are not only crucial to satisfying legal and other requirements but are also crucial to ensuring public safety as well.

Guidelines

Various agencies issue guidelines to help establish standard practices and ensure universal testing procedures. Many regulatory agencies and professional associations have published guidelines for aseptic procedures and quality control programs for pharmacy. These evolving standards cover both good manufacturing practices and quality assurance programs.

Food and Drug Administration

The Food and Drug Administration (FDA) publishes Good Manufacturing Practices (GMPs). GMPs have been practiced for many years, and these guidelines are revised as necessary. This set of standards offers guidelines for the compounding of sterile products, while another FDA document states guidelines on the manufacture of sterile products by aseptic processing. Included in these documents are quality system regulations, which will make standards consistent with quality system requirements.

The Joint Commission

The Joint Commission, formerly known as the Joint Commission on Accreditation of Healthcare Organizations (JCAHO), publishes many general standards regarding pharmaceuticals and the facilities that manufacture, store, and deliver them. Like other organizations, such as the FDA, the Joint Commission constantly revises its standards to improve compliance and keep up with the ever-evolving field of drugs and their manufacturing processes.

Through stringent inspections performed at timed intervals, the Joint Commission offers a highly respected and often necessary accreditation for health care organizations. Its focus is on the current state of health care and the potential for safer, higher-quality care. In addition to its published set of guidelines, the Joint Commission offers support to help organizations understand, participate, and comply with the accreditation process.

Centers for Disease Control and Prevention

The Centers for Disease Control and Prevention (CDC) publishes guidelines to assist in the prevention of spreading disease or infection. Since the primary goal of aseptic compounding mirrors these guidelines, it is easy to see why the CDC documents would be important to understand and put into practice. CDC guidelines also provide invaluable information for hospital environment controls, especially where infection prevention is concerned.

American Society of Health-System Pharmacists

Some of the most widely and longest recognized publications regarding quality assurance with sterile products, as well as all other pharmaceuticals and related information, are the guidelines established by the American Society of Health-System Pharmacists (ASHP). ASHP has taken an active role in producing documents addressing quality assurance. The ASHP *Guidelines on Quality Assurance for Pharmacy-Prepared Sterile Products* outlines the numerous considerations that are subjected to quality testing and assurance. It is a comprehensive document that addresses all areas impacted by quality assurance.

United States Pharmacopeia

The United States Pharmacopeia (USP) has published the first enforceable national standards for sterile compounding, USP 797. This major publication has gained the attention of numerous pharmacy regulatory entities, such as state boards of pharmacy, the JCAHO, the FDA, and many others. Agencies such as these are using USP 797 as a universal guide, while amending and revising their own current publications.

Miscellaneous

Other local, state, and national agencies also influence pharmacy practice and quality assurance activities. They may also have recommended and established guidelines such as through state boards of pharmacy. Find out what rules apply in the state where you practice, as it is extremely important that anyone who works in any area of pharmacy or related health care fields obtain copies of the preceding publications, read them, and understand their impact on the profession. Just as important is to reread these documents periodically, as edits, revisions, and amendments are suggested and made constantly.

Workplace Wisdom

Room temperature refers to 15°C–30°C.

Refrigerated temperature is 2°C–8°C.

Freezer temperature is −20°C to −10°C.

ASHP Guidelines on Quality Assurance for Pharmacy-Prepared Sterile Products

ASHP guidelines are divided into three risk levels as follows.

Risk Level 1

Risk level 1 includes products that are stored at room temperature and completely administered within 28 hours of preparation; unpreserved, sterile, and prepared for administration to more than one patient and contain suitable preservatives; or prepared by a **closed-system aseptic transfer** of sterile, nonpyrogenic, finished pharmaceuticals obtained from licensed manufacturers into sterile final containers obtained from licensed manufacturers.

Examples

Examples that fall in this category include the following: single-patient admixtures; sterile ophthalmics; syringes without preservatives used within 28 hours; batch-prefilled syringes with preservatives; and TPN solutions made by gravity transfer of carbohydrates and amino acids into an empty container with the addition of sterile additives with a needle and syringe.

Policies and Procedures

Up-to-date policies and procedures (P&Ps) for **compounding** sterile products should be available to all involved personnel. When policies are changed, they should be updated. Procedures should address personnel education, training, competency, product acquisition, storage, handling and delivery of final products, use and maintenance of facilities and equipment, garb and conduct of personnel, process validation, preparation technique, labeling, documentation, quality control, and material movement.

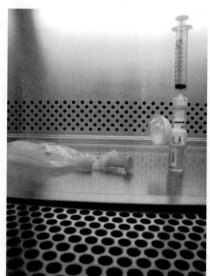

FIGURE 9-1 Closed-system transfer device

Personnel Training

All pharmacy personnel preparing sterile products should receive suitable didactic and experiential training and competency evaluation through demonstration or testing (written or practical). In addition to the P&Ps listed previously, education includes chemical, pharmaceutical, and clinical properties of drugs and current good compounding practices.

Storage and Handling Inside the Pharmacy

Solutions, drugs, supplies, and equipment must be stored according to manufacturer or USP requirements. Refrigerator and freezer temperatures as well as cleaning of the compounding areas should be documented daily. Other storage areas should be inspected regularly to ensure that temperature, light, moisture, and ventilation meet requirements. Drugs and supplies should be shelved above the floor. Expired products must be removed from active product storage areas. Personnel traffic in storage areas should be minimized. Removal of products from boxes should be done outside **controlled areas**. Disposal of used supplies should be done at least daily. Product recall procedures must permit retrieving affected products from specific involved patients.

Facilities and Equipment

Controlled areas should be separated from other operations to minimize unnecessary flow of materials and personnel through the area. Controlled areas must be clean, well lighted, and of sufficient size for sterile compounding. A sink with hot and cold water should be near, but not in, the controlled area. Controlled areas and inside equipment must be cleaned and disinfected regularly. Sterile products must be prepared in an ISO 5 environment (the critical areas) such as within a horizontal or vertical laminar airflow hood or barrier isolator. Computer entry, order processing, label generation, and record keeping should be performed outside of the critical area. The critical area must be disinfected periodically. Airflow hoods should be recertified every 6 months or when moved, and prefilters should be changed periodically. Pumps should be recalibrated according to procedure.

Garb

In controlled areas, personnel must wear low-particulate, clean clothing covers such as clean gowns or coveralls with sleeves having elastic cuffs. Hand, finger, and wrist jewelry should be minimized or eliminated. Nails should be clean and trimmed. Gloves are recommended; individuals allergic to latex rubber must wear gloves made of a suitable alternative. Head and facial hair must be covered. Masks are recommended during aseptic preparation. Personnel preparing sterile products must scrub their hands and arms with an appropriate antimicrobial skin cleanser.

Aseptic Technique and Product Preparation

Sterile products must be prepared in an ISO 5 environment. Personnel must scrub their hands and forearms for an appropriate period at the beginning of each aseptic compounding process. Eating, drinking, and smoking are prohibited in the controlled area. Talking must be minimized to reduce airborne particles. Ingredients must be determined to be stable, compatible, and appropriate for the product to be prepared according to manufacturer, USP, or scientific references. Ingredients must result in final products that meet physiologic norms as to osmolality and pH for the intended route of administration. Ingredients and containers must be inspected for defects, expiration, and integrity before use. Only materials essential for aseptic compounding must be placed in the workbench. Surfaces of ampules and vials must be disinfected before placement in the workbench. Sterile components must be arranged in the workbench to allow uninterrupted laminar airflow over critical surfaces of needles, vials, ampules, and so on. Usually only one person and one preparation are allowed in the workbench at a time. Automated devices and equipment must be cleaned, disinfected, and placed in the workbench to enable laminar airflow. Aseptic technique must be used to avoid touch contamination of critical sites of containers and ingredients. Sterile powders must be completely reconstituted.

Particles must be filtered from solutions. Needle cores must be avoided. The pharmacist must check before, during, and after preparation to verify the identity and amount of ingredients before release.

Process Validation

All personnel who prepare sterile products should pass a process validation of their aseptic technique before they prepare sterile products for patient use. Personnel competency should be reevaluated by process validation at least annually, whenever the quality assurance program yields an unacceptable result, and whenever unacceptable techniques are observed. If microbial growth is detected, the entire sterile process must be evaluated, **corrective action** taken, and the process simulation test performed again.

Handling Sterile Products Outside the Pharmacy

Sterile products must be transported so as to be protected from excesses of temperatures and light. Transit time and condition should be specified. Delivery personnel should be trained as appropriate. Pharmacists must ascertain that the end user knows how to properly store products. End users must notify pharmacists when storage conditions are exceeded or when products expire so that pharmacists can arrange safe disposal or return.

Documentation

The following must be documented according to policy, laws, and regulations: training and competency evaluation of employees, refrigerator and freezer temperature logs, certification of workbenches, and other facility quality control logs as appropriate. Pharmacists must maintain appropriate records for the compounding and dispensing of sterile products.

Expiration Dating

All sterile products must bear an appropriate expiration date. Expiration dates should be assigned based on current drug stability information and sterility considerations. The pharmacist should consider all aspects of the final product, including drug reservoir, drug concentration, and storage conditions.

Labeling

Sterile products should be labeled with at least the following information: for patient-specific products, the patient's name and other appropriate patient identification; for batch-prepared products, control or lot numbers; all solution and ingredient names, amounts, strengths, and concentrations; expiration date (and time when applicable); prescribed administration regimen; appropriate auxiliary labeling; storage requirements; identification of the responsible pharmacist; any device-specific instructions; and any additional information, in accordance with state and federal regulations. A reference number for the prescription or order may also be helpful. The label should be legible and affixed to the product so that it can be read while being administered.

End-Product Evaluations

The final product must be inspected for container leaks, integrity, solution cloudiness or phase separation, particulates in solution, appropriate solution color, and solution volume. The pharmacist must verify that the product was compounded accurately as to ingredients, quantities, containers, and reservoirs.

Risk Level 2

Risk level 2 includes products that are administered beyond 28 hours after preparation and stored at room temperature; batch-prepared without preservatives and intended for use by more than one patient; or compounded by complex or numerous manipulations of sterile ingredients obtained from licensed manufacturers by using a closed-system aseptic transfer.

Examples

Examples that fall in this category include the following: injections for use in a portable pump or reservoir over multiple days; batch-reconstituted antibiotics without preservatives; batch-prefilled syringes without preservatives; and TPN solutions mixed with an automatic compounding device.

Policies and Procedures

In addition to risk level 1 guidelines, procedures describe environmental monitoring of devices and techniques, cleaning of materials and disinfectants, equipment accuracy monitoring, limits of acceptability and corrective actions for environmental monitoring and process validation, master formula sheets and worksheets, personnel garb, lot numbers, and other quality control methods.

Personnel Training

In addition to guidelines in risk level 1, training includes assessment of competency in all types of risk level 2 procedures via process simulation. Personnel must show competency in end product testing.

Storage and Handling Inside the Pharmacy

All guidelines for risk level 1 apply.

Facilities and Equipment

In addition to risk level 1 guidelines, controlled areas must meet at least ISO 7 clean room standards. Cleaning supplies should be selected to meet **clean room** standards. The **critical area** work surface must be cleaned between batches. Floors should be disinfected daily, equipment surfaces weekly, and walls monthly. There should be environmental monitoring of air and surfaces. An anteroom of high cleanliness is desirable. Automated compounding devices must be calibrated and verified as to ensure accuracy according to procedure.

Garb

In addition to risk level 1 guidelines, gloves, gowns, and masks are required. During sterile preparation, gloves should be rinsed frequently with a suitable agent (such as 70% isopropyl alcohol) and changed when their integrity is compromised. Shoe covers are helpful in maintaining the cleanliness of the controlled area.

Aseptic Technique and Product Preparation

In addition to risk level 1 guidelines, a master worksheet containing formula, components, procedures, sample label, final evaluation, and testing is made for each product batch. A separate worksheet and lot number are used for each batch. When combining multiple sterile ingredients, a second pharmacist should verify calculations. The pharmacist should verify data entered into an automatic compounder before processing and check the end product for accuracy.

Process Validation

All risk level 1 guidelines apply, and process simulation procedures should cover all types of manipulations, products, and batch sizes that are encountered in risk level 2.

Handling Sterile Products Outside the Pharmacy

All guidelines for risk level 1 apply.

Documentation

In addition to the guidelines in risk level 1, documentation of end product testing and batch preparation records must be maintained according to policies, laws, and regulations.

Expiration Dating

All guidelines for risk level 1 apply.

Labeling

All guidelines for risk level 1 apply.

End-Product Evaluations

In addition to risk level 1 guidelines, toxic products, such as concentrated glucose and potassium chloride, should be tested for accuracy of concentration.

Risk Level 3

Risk level 3 includes products that are compounded from nonsterile ingredients or components, containers, or equipment before terminal sterilization; or prepared by combining multiple ingredients, sterile or nonsterile, by using an open-system transfer before terminal sterilization.

Examples

Examples that fall in this category include the following: alum bladder irrigation; morphine injection made from powder or tablets; TPN solutions made from dry amino acids or sterilized by final filtration; autoclaved IV solutions.

Policies and Procedures

Procedures cover every aspect of preparation of risk level 3 sterile products, so that all products have the identity, strength, quality, and purity purported for the product. Thirteen general P&Ps in addition to those in risk levels 1 and 2 are required.

Personnel Training

Operators must have specific education, training, and experience to prepare risk level 3 products. They must understand principles of good compounding practice for risk level 3 products including aseptic processing; component and end-product testing; sterilization; and selection and use of containers, equipment, and closures.

Storage and Handling Inside the Pharmacy

In addition to risk level 1 guidelines, procedures include procurement, identification, storage, handling, testing, and recall of components and finished products. Finished but untested products must be quarantined under a minimal risk for contamination or loss of identity in an identified quarantine area.

Facilities and Equipment

Products must be prepared in an ISO 5 workbench in an ISO 7 clean room, in an ISO 5 clean room, or in a suitable barrier isolator. Access to the clean room must be limited to those preparing the products who are in appropriate garb.

Methods are needed for cleaning, preparing, sterilizing, calibrating, and documenting the use of all equipment. Walls and ceilings should be disinfected weekly. All nonsterile equipment that is to come in contact with the sterilized final product should be sterilized before introduction into the clean room. An anteroom of high cleanliness (at least ISO 8) should be provided. Appropriate cleaning and disinfection of the environment and equipment are required.

Garb

In addition to risk level 1 and 2 guidelines, clean room garb must be worn inside the controlled area at all times during the preparation of risk level 3 sterile products. Attire consists of a low-shedding coverall, head cover, face mask, and shoe covers. Before donning this garb, personnel must thoroughly wash their hands and arms. Upon return to the controlled area or support area during processing, personnel should regown with clean garb.

Aseptic Technique and Product Preparation

In addition to risk level 1 and 2 guidelines, nonsterile components must meet USP standards for identity, purity, and endotoxin levels, as verified by a pharmacist. Batch master worksheets should also include comparisons of actual with anticipated yields, sterilization methods, and quarantine specifications.

Presterilized containers should be used if feasible. Final containers must be sterile and capable of maintaining product integrity throughout shelf life. Sterilization method is based on properties of the product. Final filtration methods require attention to many elements of product, filter, and filter integrity.

Process Validation

In addition to risk level 1 and 2 guidelines, written policies should be established to validate all processes (including all procedures, components, equipment, and techniques) for each risk level 3 product.

Handling Sterile Products Outside the Pharmacy

All guidelines for risk level 1 apply.

Documentation

In addition to risk level 1 and 2 guidelines, documentation for risk level 3 products must include a preparation worksheet, sterilization records if applicable, quarantine records if applicable, and end-product evaluation and testing records.

Expiration Dating

In addition to risk level 1 and 2 guidelines, there must be a reliable method for establishing all expiration dates, including laboratory testing of product stability, pyrogenicity, and chemical content when necessary.

Labeling

All guidelines for risk level 1 and 2 apply.

End-Product Evaluations

In addition to risk level 1 and 2 guidelines, the medium fill procedure should be supplemented with a program of end-product sterility testing according to a formal sampling plan. Samples should be statistically adequate to reasonably ensure that batches are sterile. A method for recalling batch products should be established if end-product testing yields unacceptable results. Each sterile preparation or batch must be laboratory tested for conformity to written specifications (such as for concentration and pyrogenicity). It is advisable to quarantine sterile products compounded from nonsterile components pending the results of end-product testing.

United States Pharmacopeia 797

USP 797 is the first enforceable set of standards that defines the responsibilities of many areas subjected to quality control and offers a virtually unquestionable view as to what is necessary for the quality control process. It is important as a pharmacy technician compounding sterile products that you understand their impact on your pharmacy career. Next, we briefly describe some of the common considerations in these documents.

Risk Levels

Compounded sterile products (CSPs) are grouped into three levels of risk depending on the potential risk of product contamination and loss of integrity and risk to patient safety. USP 797 classifies compounded sterile products as either low-risk-level, medium-risk-level, or high-risk-level CSPs. Risk levels define where a particular prepared product might be grouped based on the type of CSP, compounding processes, and environments. Each risk level has variant recommendations and guidelines as well, which aid in reducing contamination of all sorts.

Sometimes it can be confusing to decide under which risk level a specific product falls. A list of examples is provided to help clarify this so that you can understand all of the guidelines that apply. In any case, it is always acceptable to follow the most stringent guidelines. As the saying goes, better safe than sorry!

Low-Risk-Level Compounded Sterile Products

Any CSP that is prepared under the following conditions is considered a low-risk-level product:

1. With proper aseptic technique, the CSP is compounded in an ISO Class 5 or better environment using only sterile ingredients and supplies.

2. Simple compounding (transferring, measuring, and mixing) is used involving three or fewer commercially available products/packages with no more than two entries into any one sterile IV bag or vial.

3. Aseptic manipulations are limited aseptically: opening ampules, transferring liquids in syringes to sterile containers, devices, or packages, and penetrating disinfected vial stoppers.

4. Without passing a sterility test, low-risk-level CSPs, before administration, cannot be stored longer than 48 hours at controlled room temperature, 14 days refrigerated, and 45 days frozen.

Examples of low-risk CSPs include single-volume transfers of sterile dosage forms from ampules (through a sterile filter), bottles, bags, and vials using sterile syringes, needles, or other administration devices.

Low-Risk-Level Compounded Sterile Products with 12-Hour or Less Beyond-Use Date

If the ISO Class 5 PEC cannot be located within an ISO Class 7 buffer area, then the low-risk-level CSP will have only a 12-hour or less beyond-use date (BUD). Low-risk-level CSPs with a 12-hour or less BUD must meet the following criteria:

1. PECs must be certified and maintain an ISO Class 5 environment and must be in a segregated compounding area, and any sinks should be separate from the immediate area of the PEC.

2. The compounding area should not have unsealed windows or doors that connect to the outside or high-traffic areas, adjacent to construction sites, warehouses, or food preparation areas.

3. Personnel must follow USP 797 guidelines for proper cleansing and garb.

Quality Assurance for Low-Risk-Level Compounded Sterile Products

Quality assurance practices should include the following:

1. Routine disinfections and air quality testing of the DCA to minimize contamination and maintain ISO Class 5 air environment.

2. Visual confirmation that proper PPE is being used by compounding personnel.

3. Review of all compounding orders, packages, and CSPs to ensure correct medications and amounts were compounded.

4. Visual inspection of CSP to ensure that there are no leaks or particulate matter and that the labeling is correct.

5. Every person compounding low-risk level CSPs must perform a media-fill test or equivalent at least once per year. The media-fill test is used to "assess the quality of the aseptic skill of compounding personnel." The test must be performed in the ISO 5 environment, and, once begun, it must be completed without interruption. An example test would include three sets of four 5-mL aliquots of sterile soybean-casein digest medium being transferred, using the same sterile 10-mL syringe and needle, into empty, sterile, 30-mL clear vials. Sterile adhesive seals are affixed to each 30-mL vial, and the vials are incubated for a minimum of 14 days to determine if growth is present.

Medium-Risk-Level Compounded Sterile Products

Any CSP that is prepared under the following conditions is considered a medium-risk level product:

1. Multiple individual or small doses of sterile products are combined to prepare CSPs that will be administered to either multiple patients or to one patient on multiple occasions.

2. Compounding processes include complex manipulations of long duration that involve processes other than single-volume transfer.

3. Without passing a sterility test, medium-risk level CSPs, before administration, cannot be stored longer than 30 hours at controlled room temperature, 9 days refrigerated, and 45 days frozen.

Examples of medium-risk level CSPs include TPN, filling infusion devices with more than three drug products and removing air from the reservoirs, and transferring from multiple ampules or vials into one or more final container.

Quality Assurance for Medium-Risk-Level Compounded Sterile Products

Quality assurance practices should include all procedures for low-risk-level products as well as a more difficult media-fill test, which is passed at least annually. The media-fill test for medium-risk-level products includes six 100-mL aliquots of soybean-casein digest medium that are transferred using gravity into separated evacuated containers. With a pair of evacuated containers and a 10-mL syringe and 18-G needle, 5 mL are removed from one container and injected into the second container and agitated for 10 sec. After agitation, 5 mL are removed from the container and injected back into the first container. Then, 5 mL are removed from both containers and injected into a 10-mL clear, empty vial, sealed, and incubated for 14 days. This process is repeated for three pairs of evacuated containers.

High-Risk-Level Compounded Sterile Products

Any CSP that is prepared under the following conditions is considered contaminated or at a high-risk for contamination:

1. Compounding is done using nonsterile ingredients.

2. Sterile contents of commercially manufactured products, CSPs without antimicrobial preservatives, or sterile surfaces of devices/containers are exposed to air quality worse than an ISO Class 5 environment for more than 1 hour.

3. Personnel are improperly gowned.

4. Before sterilization, nonsterile water-containing products are stored for greater than 6 hours.

5. Without passing a sterility test, high-risk-level CSPs, before administration, cannot be stored longer than 24 hours at controlled room temperature, 3 days refrigerated, and 45 days frozen.

All supplies and equipment used for measuring and mixing high-risk-level products must be rinsed with sterile, pyrogen-free water and drained or dried immediately before use in high-risk compounding. All high-risk CSPs must be prefiltered with a filter not larger than 1.2 microns before sterilization. A 0.2-micron filter must be used for filtration sterilization of high-risk products in an ISO Class 5 environment.

Examples of high-risk level products include those prepared by dissolving nonsterile ingredients and nutrient powders for terminal sterilization and from measuring and mixing sterile ingredients in nonsterile devices before sterilization.

Quality Assurance for High-Risk-Level Compounded Sterile Products

Quality assurance practices should include all procedures for low-risk-level and medium-risk-level products as well as a high-risk media-fill test, which is passed at least semiannually by each person preparing high-risk-level products. A high-risk media-fill test would include dissolving 3 g of nonsterile soybean-casein digest medium in 100 mL of nonbacteriostatic water. After dissolution, 25 mL are withdrawn into three 30-mL syringes and 5 mL are transferred from each syringe into sterile empty 10-mL vials. A 0.2-micron filter is attached to each 30-mL syringe and 10 mL are transferred into three separate empty vials. This is repeated for three more vials, and all vials are sealed and incubated for 14 days.

Environmental Sampling Testing

USP 797 requires that each compounding pharmacy perform environmental sampling testing as part of their quality management program. Environmental sampling testing will occur in the following situations:

1. Upon the commissioning of new facilities and equipment

2. Following any servicing of facilities and equipment

3. As part of periodic recertification of facilities and equipment

4. In response to issues with compounded sterile products or observed improper technique of compounding personnel or if a CSP is considered a potential source of patient-related infection.

All primary engineering controls as well as the buffer and ante areas must be verified and certified for proper air quality. Certification of all equipment and compounding areas must occur at least every 6 months or whenever a PEC or room is moved, serviced, or altered.

Cleaning and Disinfecting The Compounding Area

As part of the pharmacy's quality assurance program and activities, USP 797 requires that compounding areas be cleaned and disinfected at the following minimum frequencies:

- The primary engineering control (ISO Class 5) must be cleaned and disinfected at the beginning of each shift, before each batch, at least every 30 minutes following the previous disinfection during continuous compounding activities, after spills, or when suspected contamination occurs.

- Counters, work surfaces, and floors must be cleaned and disinfected daily when no aseptic compounding is occurring.

- Walls, ceilings, and storage shelving must be cleaned and disinfected monthly.

USP recommends that all cleaning supplies (wipes, sponges, mops) be made of a nonshedding material (synthetic microfibers) and be disposed of after use. If the supplies are reused, the pharmacy must ensure that the supplies maintain their cleaning effectiveness.

Policies and Procedures

There is not a pharmacy in the United States that can operate without policies and procedures that address updating, accessibility to personnel, accuracy, standard operating procedures (SOPs), monitoring, and much more. Not only do they apply to drug processes, but single of aspect of pharmacy must also have P&Ps. Every person working in a pharmacy has the responsibility of knowing the policies and procedures that impact them in their daily routines. Workplaces carry the responsibility of providing the P&Ps and keeping them updated. Know your policies and procedures.

Personnel, Education, and Evaluation

We all know that it is important for personnel to have proper training and skills to perform their duties in a pharmacy. Because pharmacy is ever evolving, including areas of sterile products, personnel must also constantly update their skills and continue their education to stay abreast of this wealth of information. Facilities must have a process for evaluating the skills (assessment) and knowledge of their personnel to ensure that they are competent in their practice. Well-educated and well-trained professionals are key to minimizing risks and errors. This is a never-ending process that continues throughout your pharmacy career.

Storage and Handling Inside and Outside the Pharmacy

It is extremely important how medications are packaged, prepared, and delivered. Once a final product is presented, it can easily be compromised if it is not stored or handled properly. For example, suppose that an IV solution that needs to be refrigerated is not placed in a refrigerator. Stability and contamination ensue, and the product is no longer safe to use. In addition to the waste that occurs, how can we ensure that the contaminated product does not reach the patient? The same can be said of a preparation that is not done properly in an aseptic manner. Before the final product is delivered to the patient, it has already been compromised and could do great harm if the error goes undetected.

Facilities and Equipment

Great care should be taken when designing a facility that will be performing aseptic compounding. All areas where actual compounding takes place, in particular, are held to extremely high standards. As you have read in previous chapters, anterooms, critical areas, clean rooms, and many other areas fall under this category. In addition, all equipment and supplies used in aseptic compounding facilities must be installed properly, used properly, maintained, and monitored.

Aseptic Technique, Product Preparation, and Garb

Much emphasis is placed on the actual processes that take place during manufacturing. Any process that requires constant evaluation and improvement has many checkpoints. Major focus in this area is on the prevention of microbial contamination. All of the things considered here involve ingredients, components, proper gowning, and all supplies used in aseptic compounding.

Process Validation

The FDA defines process validation as "establishing documented evidence which provides a high degree of assurance that a specific process will consistently produce a product meeting its pre-determined specifications and quality characteristics." Each stage in the validation of the overall process should proceed in accordance with a preestablished and formally approved, detailed, written protocol or series of related protocols. Personnel should be assessed as to their competency in performing and understanding these protocols. In addition, controls should be in place to prevent unauthorized changes to the processes or protocols, especially in the absence of relevant data. There are numerous requirements to the process validations, such as identification numbers and specific methodology on how to obtain and test samples. Nothing is exempt from a process validation, including hand washing, aseptic technique, storage, and training. Even reevaluating the validation process is subject to this control measure. Also included here are guidelines for corrective measures when integrity falters. A procedure must be in place to correct situations—everything from discovery, reporting, and data collection to corrective actions.

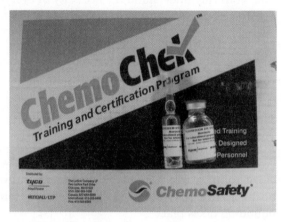

FIGURE 9-2 ChemoCheck validation test kit

End-Product Evaluation

After all of the other considerations that have been addressed, it is time for the final check. This is known as the end-product evaluation. Pharmacy technicians may think that this is the pharmacist's final check, but that is only a small part. Also included are inspections, more specifically with periodic sampling of batches manufactured under the exact same conditions and then tested.

Documentation and Labeling

Without a doubt, pharmacy requires extensive documentation of all sorts. All products dispensed must be labeled, and all components used must be identified. Every piece of equipment must have records. A pharmacy may have several methods or forms for different documentation needs. For example, SOPs illustrate how a product is made or processed. Having an SOP for each procedure not only helps to ensure that each person about to prepare a product knows the correct procedure, but it also ensures consistency with each preparation.

A crucial part of any IV or chemotherapy preparation is documentation. Documentation is a record of patient information, product preparation, label information, and any other important information regarding the product or how it was made. For each product made for each patient, there must be documentation that includes information about the patient, such as patient diagnosis, IV regimen, dosages, body surface area, lab values, and other pertinent information. Another part of this record is a worksheet that has information regarding the preparation and final product, such as ingredients, preparation or process, labeling, storage and handling information, expiration date, batch/lot identifying numbers, warnings, and other miscellaneous information.

Controlled substances require even more documentation than noncontrolled substances. Accurate and proper record keeping and documentation are essential and require strict guidelines to ensure the origin of all components, the process performed, and all other things mentioned in this chapter.

Each facility may have its own forms, but the fundamentals are the same. Final products and processes have certain information such as that described previously, which must be included and kept for a time period to be determined based on the information, laws and regulations, and facility policy.

It is highly important that as a sterile-products-compounding pharmacy technician, you become familiar with and understand how to fill out required documentation forms completely and accurately. This is an area of pharmacy that must not be overlooked and is often scrutinized during compliance inspections.

CONCLUSION

Quality assurance of sterile products and procedures is very complex and requires acute awareness of every aspect of pharmaceuticals and constant research to stay abreast of the area. Each step of the manufacturing and compounding process must be controlled to ensure that the finished product meets all quality and design specifications. If you understand **quality control** measures, however, you truly understand the necessity of everything you do. To recap, **quality assurance** involves the following:

- Personnel training and competency
- Various quality assurance steps
- Environmental control and monitoring

- Quality testing of compounded dosage forms
- Personnel aseptic technique evaluation
- Determination of product risk
- Storage and beyond-use dating
- Standard operating procedures

Many publications offer guidelines to follow in order to prevent contamination and maintain and improve safety for the patient. USP 797 expands on many previously written documents and helps clarify specific measures that pharmacies must take to sustain a national standard consistent with all practices.

CHAPTER TERMS

clean room a room in which the concentration of airborne particles is controlled and where aseptic compounding takes place

closed-system aseptic transfer the movement of sterile products from one container to another in which the containers, closure system, and transfer devices remain intact throughout the entire transfer process

compounding the mixing of ingredients to prepare a medication for patient use

controlled area the area designated for preparing sterile products; also called the clean room, in which the laminar airflow hood is located

corrective action actions taken when the results of monitoring indicate a loss of control or when predetermined action levels are exceeded

critical area any area in the controlled area where products and other materials are exposed to the environment

process validation microbiological simulation of an aseptic process with growth medium processed in a manner similar to the processing of the product and with the same container or closure system

quality assurance the set of activities used to ensure that the processes used in the preparation of sterile drug products lead to products that meet predetermined standards of quality

quality control the set of testing activities used to determine that the ingredients, components (such as containers), and final sterile products prepared meet predetermined requirements for purity, nonpyrogenicity, and sterility

CHAPTER REVIEW QUESTIONS

MULTIPLE CHOICE

1. Right medication, dose, route, time, patient, technique, and documentation are referred to as _____.
   a. the patient bill of rights
   b. the seven rights
   c. right medication administration
   d. right place, right time
   e. distribution rights

2. Compromising a quality control measure may result in what devastating effect?
   a. termination from a job
   b. a change in the uniforms that are worn
   c. microbial contamination
   d. bad documentation
   e. changed expiration dates

3. _____ provides accreditation to facilities that have passed strict guidelines relating to patient care.
   a. The Food and Drug Administration
   b. The Drug Enforcement Agency
   c. The United States Pharmacopeia
   d. The Joint Commission
   e. HIPAA

4. _____ is the first enforceable national published standards regarding sterile products.
   a. HIPAA 797
   b. USP 297
   c. JCAHO 123
   d. CDC 597
   e. USP 797

5. What three criteria are involved in ensuring quality for personnel performing aseptic compounding?

   a. dressing, hand washing, continuing education
   b. training, education, attendance
   c. needle manipulation, hood cleaning, competency
   d. competency, training, education
   e. experience, didactic training, ability

6. Sampling finished products and testing for integrity falls under which topic of quality assurance?

   a. process validation
   b. end-product evaluation
   c. equipment and
   d. labeling
   e. storage and ha

7. For aseptic techni
   low-risk level, the
   environment.

   a. ISO Class 3
   b. ISO Class 5
   c. ISO Class 6
   d. ISO Class 7
   e. ISO Class 8

8. For aseptic tech
   high-risk level,
   environment.

   a. ISO Class 3
   b. ISO Class 5
   c. ISO Class 6
   d. ISO Class
   e. ISO Class

9. Environmenta
   the commissi
   facilities and
   servicing of s

   a. true
   b. false

10. Which of th
    to enforce (

    a. United S
    b. NABP
    c. Food and Drug Administration
    d. Joint Commission on Accreditation of Healthcare Organizations
    e. Drug Enforcement Agency

11. A low-risk-level product can be stored for a maximum of _____ at room temperature.

    a. 16 hr
    b. 20 hr

c. 24 hr
d. 30 hr
e. 48 hr

12. A high-risk-level product can be stored for a maximum of _____ at room temperature.

    a. 16 hr
    b. 20 hr
    c. 24 hr
    d. 30 hr
    e. 48 hr

13. An example of a high-risk-level is _____.

    a. CSP compounded using a single volume transfer of drug
       CSP compounded using multiple volume transfers of drug
       TPN
       CSP compounded using nonsterile equipment
       none of the above

    example of a medium-risk-level product is _____.

       CSP compounded using a single volume transfer of drug
       CSP compounded using multiple volume transfers of drug
       TPN
       CSP compounded using nonsterile equipment
       none of the above

    ECs should be cleaned and disinfected _____.

       daily
       monthly
       at the beginning of each shift and at least every 30 min thereafter
       after each batch
       both c and d

    Which of the following compounding areas should be cleaned at least monthly?

       PEC
       walls
       floors
       counters
       both c and d

    Which of the following compounding areas should be cleaned at least on a daily basis?

    a. PEC
    b. walls
    c. floors
    d. counters
    e. both c and d

Appendix A
Terminology and Abbreviations

Terminology

acid   describes a substance that increases the concentration of hydrogen ions (lowers the pH); an acidic substance is called an acid

additive   any drug or component added to an IV solution

admixture   an IV solution with at least one medication added to it

aerosolization   a process resulting in a suspension of small particles (liquid or powder) in the air

albumin   the protein of the highest concentration in plasma

alkaline   describes a substance that decreases the concentration of hydrogen ions (raises the pH); an alkaline substance is called a base

amino acid   any organic acid containing one or more amino groups ($-NH_2$) and one or more carboxyl groups ($-COOH$); amino acids are the building blocks of proteins

ampule   a sealed glass container containing sterile injectable medication

ante area   an ISO Class 8 or better area where personnel hand washing and garbing procedures, staging of components, order entry, compounded sterile product labeling, and other high–particulate-generating activities are performed. It is a low-particulate room, which means that it should not contain paper, boxes, or high-particulate matter. Food and drink should not be allowed in this room.

antibacterial   an agent that destroys bacteria or inhibits their growth or reproduction

antibiotic   a substance produced by a living organism capable of killing or inhibiting the growth of another microorganism (example: penicillin)

anticoagulant   an agent that prevents or delays the clotting of blood (example: heparin)

antimicrobial   an agent or action that kills or inhibits the growth of microorganisms

antineoplastic   a drug intended to inhibit or prevent the maturation and proliferation of neoplasms that may become malignant

asepsis   prevention of microbial contamination of living tissues or sterile materials by excluding, removing, or killing microorganisms

aseptic   free from infection or septic material; sterile

aseptic technique   the method used to manipulate sterile products so that they remain sterile

autoclave   a steam sterilizer consisting of a metal chamber constructed to withstand the pressure that is required to raise the temperature of steam to the level required for sterilization

bacteriocidal   an agent capable of killing bacteria

bacteriostatic   capable of inhibiting the growth or reproduction of bacteria

barrel   the part of a syringe that is marked with calibrations to designate the amount of liquid it contains

batch preparation   the compounding of multiple sterile product units in a single process by the same individuals during one time period

bevel   the tip of the needle, which is slanted to prevent coring when inserting it into a rubber diaphragm

beyond-use date (BUD)   the date or time after which a compounded sterile product should not be stored or transported

biological safety cabinet (BSC)   a type of hood in which chemotherapy drugs are compounded

bolus   an initial dose of medication or solution; usually a dose higher than the maintenance dose; also called loading dose

buffer area   an area where the primary engineering control is physically located

carcinogenic   producing a malignant new growth that arises from the epithelium, which is found in skin or, more commonly, the lining of body organs

central line   IV access directly through a central blood vessel

chemo bags   bags in which completed chemo intravenous bags or syringes are placed for transport; they can also be brought into the BSC for trash disposal to help minimize movement in and out of the BSC

chemo mat   an absorbent mat placed in the BSC; the intravenous tech should compound cytotoxic agents on top of the chemo mat in case of any spills

chemo pin   a pin that is very similar to a dispensing pin; however, the vented area of a chemo pin has a special filter to reduce any aerosolization of chemotherapy product

chemotherapy   treatment of cancer with drugs (chemicals)

clean room   a room in which the concentration of airborne particles is controlled to meet a specified airborne particulate cleanliness class

closed-system transfer   the movement of sterile products from one container to another in which the containers, closure system, and transfer devices remain intact throughout the entire transfer process

compatibility   a feature of two or more components that can be mixed with each other without any physical and/or chemical stability problems in the admixture

compounding   the mixing of ingredients to prepare a medication for patient use

contamination   the act of introducing a harmful substance

continuous infusion   larger volume of solution (250 mL or more) infused at a constant rate over a longer administration time

controlled area   the area designated for preparing sterile products; also called the clean room, in which the laminar airflow hood is located

coring   the breaking off a part of the rubber stopper of a vial or container due to an improper needle stick; the cored part of the rubber stopper is usually pushed into the vial or container

corrective action   actions taken when the results of monitoring indicate a loss of control or when predetermined action levels are exceeded

critical area   any area in the controlled area where products and other materials are exposed to the environment

cytotoxic   describes chemicals that are directly toxic to cells, preventing their reproduction or growth

decompensate   to fail to maintain adequate flow or amounts

desiccation   the act of dehydrating or removing water content

diluent   a liquid added to a solution to reduce its concentration

disinfectant   an agent that is intended to kill or remove pathogenic microorganisms

electrolytes   primary elements necessary for the proper function of the tissues of the human body (examples: potassium, sodium, magnesium)

enteral   a method of nutrient delivery in which medication is given directly into the gastrointestinal tract

enzymes   complex proteins that cause a specific chemical change in other substances without being changed themselves

epidural (EP)   an injection of medication or fluid directly into the epidural space or the space between the spinal cord and vertebrae

germicidal   describes an agent that kills pathogenic microorganisms

gravity filling   the free flow, due to gravity, of liquid from a container placed on a higher level to another one placed below it

HEPA filter   (high-efficiency particulate air) a filter capable of retaining 99.97% of all particles 0.3 micron or larger in diameter

heparin   a sulfated mucopolysaccharide, found in granules of mast cells, that inhibits the action of thrombin on fibrinogen by potentiating antithrombins, thereby interfering with the blood clotting cascade; platelet factor IV will neutralize heparin

hub   the bottom part of the needle, which is used to attach the needle to the syringe; it must remain sterile

hyperglycemia   too high a level of glucose

hypertonic   describes a solution with a greater concentration of dissolved substances than that of body fluids or blood cells; a solution with a concentration greater than 0.9% saline or greater than 5% dextrose; any solution with a greater osmotic pressure than that of human blood serum

hypoglycemia   too low a level of glucose

hypotonic   describes a solution with a lower concentration of dissolved substances than that of body fluids or blood cells; a solution with a concentration less than 0.9% saline or less than 5% dextrose; any solution with a lower osmotic pressure than that of human blood serum

immunocompromised   a condition in which the immune system is not functioning normally

infusion   the slow administration of mediation or solution via a parenteral route of administration

intramuscular (IM)   an injection deep into a large muscle mass, such as the buttocks, thighs, and upper arms

intrathecal   an injection of medication or fluid directly into the intrathecal space surrounding the spinal cord

intravenous (IV)   an injection directly into the bloodstream

intravenous piggyback (IVPB)   a small-volume IV fluid that normally has medication added

intravenous push (IVP)   small-volume injection (10 mL or less) directly from a syringe into the vein

irrigation   a solution used for washing

iso-osmotic   having the same osmotic pressure

isotonic   describes a solution in which body cells can be bathed without net flow of water across the semipermeable cell membrane; also describes a solution with the same tonicity as another solution

laminar airflow hood   a specialized apparatus for preparing sterile pharmaceuticals, contains a special HEPA filter designed to provide a pathogen- and pyrogen-free workspace

loading dose   an initial dose of a drug that is used to achieve a desired drug level

lyophilized   describes a medication that comes in the form of a freeze-dried powder; it must be reconstituted before use

malignant   tending to become progressively worse and to result in death

media-fill test   a test used to qualify aseptic techniques by compounding personnel or processes and to ensure that the processes used are able to produce sterile products without contamination

metathesis   a mere change in place of a morbid substance, without removal from the body

narcotic   a drug that is potentially addicting; sometimes used to relieve pain; a controlled substance

negative pressure   occurs when the pressure outside a vial or bottle is greater than the pressure inside it, creating a partial vacuum; negative pressure is used when working with ceftazidime, chemotherapy drugs, mannitol, and any other drugs as instructed, as too much pressure will cause these drugs to leak from the vial

neonate   a newborn baby

osmolality   the concentration of solute in a solution per unit of solvent; commonly expressed as milliosmoles per kilogram

osmolarity   the concentration of solute in a solution per unit of solution; commonly expressed as milliosmoles per liter

osmosis   the tendency of a solvent to pass through a semipermeable membrane (such as the cell wall) into a solution of higher concentration to equalize concentrations on both sides of the membrane

parenteral injection   administration via injection

particulates   small matter

pathogen   disease-causing organisms such as bacteria, fungus, and viruses

peripheral line   IV access through peripheral veins in the arms, legs, hands, or feet

permeability   the property or state of being penetrable

phlebitis   inflammation of a vein

positive pressure   occurs when the pressure inside a vial or bottle is greater than the pressure outside it; it is sometimes helpful to use positive pressure when drawing up large volumes of solutions; the plunger will drift back by a volume equal to the amount of air added, thereby requiring less energy to withdraw fluid

preservative   any additive intended to extend the content, stability, or sterility of active ingredients

process validation   microbiological simulation of an aseptic process with growth medium processed in a manner similar to the processing of the product and with the same container or closure system

protocol   the standard plan for a course of medical treatment

pyrogen   a substance that produces fever

quality assurance   the set of activities used to ensure that the processes used in the preparation of sterile drug products lead to products that meet predetermined standards of quality

quality control   the set of testing activities used to determine that the ingredients, components (such as containers), and final sterile products prepared meet predetermined requirements for identity, purity, nonpyrogenicity, and sterility

reconstitute   to add a diluent to a vial to create a liquid

renal failure   loss of the kidneys' ability to excrete wastes, concentrate urine, and conserve electrolytes

sanitization   a process that reduces microbial contamination to a low level by the use of cleaning solutions, hot water, or chemical disinfectants

sepsis   the presence of organisms in the blood

shadowing   the act of blocking airflow in the BSC

single-dose vial (SDV)   a vial that contains no preservatives; once the container is entered, contaminants may have been introduced and the container is no longer sterile

solute   any substance that dissolves another substance

specific gravity   the weight of a substance compared (as a ratio) with that of an equal volume of water

sterility   the state of being free from microorganisms

sticky mats   mats placed on the floor in the entrance from the anteroom to the clean room; the mats have multiple layers of sticky sheets that can be removed one layer at a time; the mats remove any particulates that may be carried into the clean room on the bottoms of the feet

subcutaneous (SC, SQ, subq)   an injection into the fatty subcutaneous tissue of the skin

teratogenic   tending to produce anomalies of formation

vial   a small bottle or container that holds products such as injectable medications

yellow hazardous disposal containers   containers used to dispose of hazardous medications and the equipment used to compound them; these containers require special disposal

Appendix B
Common Intravenous Medications

Alphabetical—Generic Name

GENERIC NAME	BRAND NAME	USE
acetazolamide Na	Diamox	antiglaucoma; anticonvulsant; diuretic; urinary alkalinizer
acyclovir	Zovirax	antiviral
aminophylline	Theophylline	bronchodilator; respiratory stimulant
aminodarone HCl	Cordarone	antiarrhythmic
atracurium besylate	Tacrium	skeletal muscle relaxant
aztreonam	Azactam	antibiotic
cefazolin Na	Ancef; Kefzol	antibiotic
cefoperazone Na	Cefobid	antibiotic
cefotaxime Na	Claforan	antibiotic
cefotetan	Cefotan	antibiotic
cefoxitin Na	Mefoxin	antibiotic
ceftazidime	Ceptaz; Fortaz	antibiotic
ceftizoxime Na	Cefizox	antibiotic
ceftriaxone Na	Rocephin	antibiotic
cefuroxime Na	Kefurox; Zinacef	antibiotic
cimetidine	Tagamet	antiulcer; gastric acid inhibitor
clindamycin	Cleocin	antibacterial; antiprotozoal
dexamethasone	Decadron	antiinflammatory; antiemetic; immunosuppressant
dobutamine HCl	Dobutrex	inotropic agent; cardiac stimulant
dopamine HCl	Intropin	inotropic agent; cardiac stimulant; vasopressor
doxycycline	Vibramycin; Doxy	antibacterial; antiprotozoal; antimalarial
epinephrine HCl	Adrenalin Chloride	cardiac stimulant; bronchodilator; antiallergic; vasopressor
famotidine	Pepcid	antiulcer; gastric acid inhibitor
furosemide	Lasix	diuretic; antihypertensive; antihypercalcemic
gentamicin	Garamycin	antibacterial
heparin Na	Hep-Lock; HepFlush	anticoagulant
hydromorphone HCl	Dilaudid	narcotic analgesic
imipenem-cilastatin	Primaxin	antibacterial
isoproterenol	Isuprel	cardiac stimulant; bronchodilator; antiarrhythmic
kanamycin	Kantrex	antibacterial
labetalol	Normodyne; Trandate	alpha/beta-adrenergic blocking agent; antihypertensive
lidocaine	Xylocaine	antiarrhythmic
meperidine HCl	Demerol	narcotic analgesic; anesthesia adjunct

GENERIC NAME	BRAND NAME	USE
meropenem	Merrem	antibacterial
metoclopramide HCl	Reglan	gastrointestinal stimulant; antiemetic
morphine	Astramorph; Duramorph	narcotic analgesic; anesthesia adjunct
nafcillin Na	Nafcil; Nallpen	antibacterial
nitroglycerin	Nitro-Bid; Tridil	antianginal; antihypertensive; vasodilator
norepinephrine	Levophed	vasopressor
ondansetron HCl	Zofran	antiemetic
oxacillin Na	Bactocill; Prostaphlin	antibacterial
pancuronium	Pavulon	neuromuscular blocking agent; anesthesia adjunct
pentobarbital Na	Nembutal Na	barbiturate; sedative; anticonvulsant
piperacillin/tazobactam	Zosyn	antibacterial
prochlorperazine	Compazine	antiemetic; antipsychotic
promethazine	Phenergan	antiemetic; sedative
propranolol	Inderal	beta-adrenergic blocking agent; antiarrhythmic
ranitidine	Zantac	H_2 antagonist; antiulcer agent; gastric acid inhibitor
succinylcholine	Anectine	neuromuscular blocking agent; anesthesia adjunct
thiopental	Pentothal Na	barbiturate; general anesthetic; anticonvulsant
thymoglobulin	Antithymocyte Globulin	immunosuppressant
tigecycline	Tygacil	antibiotic
tranexamic acid	Cyklokapron	antifibrinolytic; antihemorrhagic
warfarin	Coumadin	anticoagulant
zidovudine	Retrovir	antiviral

Alphabetical—Brand Name

BRAND NAME	GENERIC NAME	USE
Adrenalin Chloride	epinephrine HCl	cardiac stimulant; bronchodilator; antiallergic; vasopressor
Ancef; Kefzol	cefazolin Na	antibacterial
Anectine	succinylcholine	neuromuscular blocking agent; anesthesia adjunct
Antithymocyte Globulin	thymoglobulin	immunosuppressant
Astramorph; Duramorph	morphine	narcotic analgesic; anesthesia adjunct
Azactam	aztreonam	antibacterial
Bactocill; Prostaphlin	oxacillin Na	antibacterial
Cefizox	ceftizoxime Na	antibacterial
Cefobid	cefoperazone Na	antibacterial
Cefotan	cefotetan	antibacterial
Ceptaz; Fortaz	ceftazidime	antibacterial
Claforan	cefotaxime Na	antibacterial
Cleocin	clindamycin	antibacterial; antiprotozoal

BRAND NAME	GENERIC NAME	USE
Compazine	prochlorperazine	antiemetic; antipsychotic
Coumadin	warfarin	anticoagulant
Cyklokapron	tranexamic acid	antifibrinolytic; antihemorrhagic
Decadron	dexamethasone	antiinflammatory; antiemetic; immunosuppressant
Demerol	meperidine HCl	narcotic analgesic; anesthesia adjunct
Diamox	acetazolamide Na	antiglaucoma; anticonvulsant; diuretic; urinary alkalinizer
Dilaudid	hydromorphone HCl	narcotic analgesic
Dobutrex	dobutamine HCl	inotropic agent; cardiac stimulant
Garamycin	gentamicin	antibacterial
Hep-Lock; Hep-Flush	heparin Na	anticoagulant
Inderal	propranolol	beta-adrenergic blocking agent; antiarrhythmic
Intropin	dopamine HCl	inotropic agent; cardiac stimulant; vasopressor
Isuprel	isoproterenol	cardiac stimulant; bronchodilator; antiarrhythmic
Kantrex	kanamycin	antibacterial
Kefurox; Zinacef	cefuroxime Na	antibacterial
Lasix	furosemide	diuretic; antihypertensive; antihypercalcemic
Levophed	norepinephrine	vasopressor
Mefoxin	cefoxitin Na	antibacterial
Merrem	meropenem	antibacterial
Nafcil; Nallpen	nafcillin Na	antibacterial
Nembutal Na	pentobarbital Na	barbiturate; sedative; anticonvulsant
Nitro-Bid; Tridil	nitroglycerin	antianginal; antihypertensive; vasodilator
Normodyne; Trandate	labetalol	alpha/beta-adrenergic blocking agent; antihypertensive
Pavulon	pancuronium	neuromuscular blocking agent; anesthesia adjunct
Pentothal Na	thiopental	barbiturate; general anesthetic; anticonvulsant
Pepcid	famotidine	antiulcer; gastric acid inhibitor
Phenergan	promethazine	antiemetic; sedative
Primaxin	imipenem-cilastatin	antibacterial
Reglan	metoclopramide HCl	gastrointestinal stimulant; antiemetic
Retrovir	zidovudine	antiviral
Rocephin	ceftriaxone Na	antibacterial
Tagamet	cimetidine	antiulcer; gastric acid inhibitor
Theophylline	aminophylline	bronchodilator; respiratory stimulant
Vibramycin; Doxy	doxycycline	antibacterial; antiprotozoal; antimalarial
Xylocaine	lidocaine	antiarrhythmic
Zantac	ranitidine	H_2 antagonist; antiulcer agent; gastric acid inhibitor
Zofran	ondansetron HCl	antiemetic
Zosyn	piperacillin/tazobactam	antibacterial
Zovirax	acyclovir	antiviral

Appendix C
Training and Validation Forms

Aseptic Technique Training Log

Student Name

Date

Start Time

End Time

Contact Hour(s)

Location

Trainer's Name

Trainer's Lic. #

State of License

Daytime Phone (trainer)

Skill(s) Covered

By signing below, I validate that the information listed above is complete and fully accurate.

_____   _____   _____   _____
Student Signature   Date   Trainer Signature   Date

FIGURE C-1

140

Aseptic Technique Training Log

Student Name

Date

Start Time

End Time

Contact Hour(s)

Location

Trainer's Name

Trainer's Lic. #

State of License

Daytime Phone
(trainer)

Skill(s) Covered

By signing below, I validate that the information listed above is complete and fully accurate.

_____   _____
Student Signature   Date   Trainer Signature   Date

FIGURE C-2

Aseptic Technique Training Log

Student Name	
Date	
Start Time	
End Time	
Contact Hour(s)	
Location	
Trainer's Name	
Trainer's Lic. #	
State of License	
Daytime Phone (trainer)	
Skill(s) Covered	

By signing below, I validate that the information listed above is complete and fully accurate.

Student Signature	Date	Trainer Signature	Date

FIGURE C-3

Aseptic Technique Training Log

Student Name

Date

Start Time

End Time

Contact Hour(s)

Location

Trainer's Name

Trainer's Lic. #

State of License

Daytime Phone
(trainer)

Skill(s) Covered

By signing below, I validate that the information listed above is complete and fully accurate.

_____   _____
Student Signature   Date   Trainer Signature   Date

FIGURE C-4

Aseptic Technique Training Log

Student Name

Date

Start Time

End Time

Contact Hour(s)

Location

Trainer's Name

Trainer's Lic. #

State of License

Daytime Phone
(trainer)

Skill(s) Covered

By signing below, I validate that the information listed above is complete and fully accurate.

| Student Signature | Date | Trainer Signature | Date |

Aseptic Technique Training Log

Student Name

Date

Start Time

End Time

Contact Hour(s)

Location

Trainer's Name

Trainer's Lic. #

State of License

Daytime Phone
(trainer)

Skill(s) Covered

By signing below, I validate that the information listed above is complete and fully accurate.

_____   _____   _____   _____
Student Signature   Date   Trainer Signature   Date

FIGURE C-6

Aseptic Technique Training Log

Student Name	
Date	
Start Time	
End Time	
Contact Hour(s)	
Location	
Trainer's Name	
Trainer's Lic. #	
State of License	
Daytime Phone (trainer)	
Skill(s) Covered	

By signing below, I validate that the information listed above is complete and fully accurate.

_____   _____
Student Signature   Date   Trainer Signature   Date

Aseptic Technique Training Log

Student Name

Date

Start Time

End Time

Contact Hour(s)

Location

Trainer's Name

Trainer's Lic. #

State of License

Daytime Phone
(trainer)

Skill(s) Covered

By signing below, I validate that the information listed above is complete and fully accurate.

Student Signature   Date   Trainer Signature   Date

FIGURE C-8

Aseptic Technique Training Log

Student Name

Date

Start Time

End Time

Contact Hour(s)

Location

Trainer's Name

Trainer's Lic. #

State of License

Daytime Phone
(trainer)

Skill(s) Covered

By signing below, I validate that the information listed above is complete and fully accurate.

_____   _____
Student Signature   Date   Trainer Signature   Date

FIGURE C-9

Aseptic Technique Training Log

Student Name

Date

Start Time

End Time

Contact Hour(s)

Location

Trainer's Name

Trainer's Lic. #

State of License

Daytime Phone
(trainer)

Skill(s) Covered

By signing below, I validate that the information listed above is complete and fully accurate.

_____   Date   _____   Date
Student Signature   Trainer Signature

FIGURE C-10

Process Validation Record

Aseptic Hand Washing Technique

Student Name: _____   Date: _____

PROCEDURE	Yes	No
Removed all jewelry, watches, and objects up to the elbow		
Did not have on acrylic nails or nail polish		
Started water and adjusted to the appropriate temperature		
Avoided unnecessary splashing during process		
Used sufficient disinfecting agent/cleanser		
Cleaned all four surfaces of each finger		
Cleaned all surfaces of hands, wrists, and arms up to the elbows in a circular motion		
Did not touch the sink, faucet, or other objects that could contaminate hands		
Rinsed off all soap residue		
Rinsed hands, holding them upright and allowing water to drip to the elbow		
Did not turn off water until hands were completely dry		
Turned water off with a clean, dry, lint-free paper towel		
Did not touch the faucet while turning off the water		

By signing below, I certify that the student has demonstrated 100% competency at the above task.

_____
Trainer Name (printed)

_____
Trainer Signature

_____   _____
Trainer Daytime Phone   Trainer's License #

_____   _____
Date   State Licensed

FIGURE C-11   Copyright © NPTA. All rights reserved.

Process Validation Record

Horizonal Laminar Airflow Hood

Student Name: _____   Date: _____

PROCEDURE	Yes	No
Hood was turned on and running at least 30 min prior to preparation		
Followed proper hand-washing procedure and technique		
Wore appropriate apparel		
Used clean, sterile gauze/sponge and plenty of disinfectant to clean the hood		
Cleaned the IV pole first (if applicable)		
Cleaned the sides of the hood second, starting at the top and working side to side with overlapping strokes		
Cleaned the work surface last, starting at the back and working side to side with overlapping strokes		
Did not contaminate previously cleaned surfaces		
Did not block airflow from HEPA filter		
Did not utilize outer 6 in. of the hood opening		
Properly stood outside the hood without allowing the head to enter the inside		
Knew that hood certification is every six months, if moved, or if damaged		
Knew that prefilters should be changed monthly		

By signing below, I certify that the student has demonstrated 100% competency at the above task.

_____
Trainer Name (printed)

_____
Trainer Signature

_____   _____
Trainer Daytime Phone   Trainer's License #

_____   _____
Date   State Licensed

FIGURE C-12

Process Validation Record

Vertical Laminar Airflow Hood

Student Name: _____ Date: _____

PROCEDURE	Yes	No
Hood was turned on and running at least 30 min prior to preparation		
Followed proper hand-washing procedure and technique		
Wore appropriate apparel		
Used clean, sterile gauze/sponge and plenty of disinfectant to clean the hood		
Cleaned the IV pole first (if applicable)		
Cleaned the sides of the hood second, starting at the top and working side to side with overlapping strokes		
Cleaned the back wall and inside the glass shield, starting at the top and working up and down with overlapping strokes		
Cleaned the work surface last, starting at the back and working side to side with overlapping strokes		
Did not contaminate previously cleaned surfaces		
Did not lower the glass shield more than 8 in. from the work surface prior to preparation		
Did not block airflow from HEPA filter or air intake grills at any time		
Did not utilize outer 6 in. of the hood opening		

By signing below, I certify that the student has demonstrated 100% competency at the above task.

_____
Trainer Name (printed)

_____
Trainer Signature

_____
Trainer Daytime Phone

_____
Date

_____
Trainer's License #

_____
State Licensed

FIGURE C-13

Process Validation Record

Ampule Preparation

Student Name: _____   Date: _____

PROCEDURE	Yes	No
Followed proper hand-washing procedure and technique		
Wore appropriate apparel		
Followed proper procedure and technique in cleaning the hood		
Performed all necessary calculations correctly prior to drug preparation		
Brought the correct drugs and concentrations into the hood for preparation		
Brought the correct supplies into the hood prior to preparation		
Inspected all products for particulate matter/contamination prior to use		
Cleared ampule neck of fluid before breaking		
Cleaned ampule neck correctly before breaking		
Wrapped ampule neck correctly before breaking		
Broke ampule correctly		
Attached filter device to syringe correctly		
Draw up ampule correctly, without spilling contents		
Removed filter needle and replaced it with new needle prior to injecting final container		
Drew up the correct amount of drug and checked measurement prior to injecting into container		
Cleaned additive port on final container prior to injecting drug		
Did not core or puncture side of additive port when adding drug to the final container		
Properly mixed contents of container and inspected for incompatibilities or particulate matter		
Properly sealed additive port of container		
Did not contaminate the needle or syringe during preparation		
Did not contaminate the hood		
Did not block airflow from HEPA filter or air intake grills at any time		
Did not utilize outer 6 in. of the hood opening		
Properly discarded all waste, including sharps		

By signing below, I certify that the student has demonstrated 100% competency at the above task.

_____

Trainer Name (printed)

_____

Trainer Signature

_____   _____

Trainer Daytime Phone   Trainer's License #

_____   _____

Date   State Licensed

FIGURE C-14

Process Validation Record

Ampule Preparation

Student Name: _____   Date: _____

PROCEDURE	Yes	No
Followed proper hand-washing procedure and technique		
Wore appropriate apparel		
Followed proper procedure and technique in cleaning the hood		
Performed all necessary calculations correctly prior to drug preparation		
Brought the correct drugs and concentrations into the hood for preparation		
Brought the correct supplies into the hood prior to preparation		
Inspected all products for particulate matter/contamination prior to use		
Cleared ampule neck of fluid before breaking		
Cleaned ampule neck correctly before breaking		
Wrapped ampule neck correctly before breaking		
Broke ampule correctly		
Attached filter device to syringe correctly		
Draw up ampule correctly, without spilling contents		
Removed filter needle and replaced it with new needle prior to injecting final container		
Drew up the correct amount of drug and checked measurement prior to injecting into container		
Cleaned additive port on final container prior to injecting drug		
Did not core or puncture side of additive port when adding drug to the final container		
Properly mixed contents of container and inspected for incompatibilities or particulate matter		
Properly sealed additive port of container		
Did not contaminate the needle or syringe during preparation		
Did not contaminate the hood		
Did not block airflow from HEPA filter or air intake grills at any time		
Did not utilize outer 6 in. of the hood opening		
Properly discarded all waste, including sharps		

By signing below, I certify that the student has demonstrated 100% competency at the above task.

_____

Trainer Name (printed)

_____

Trainer Signature

_____   _____

Trainer Daytime Phone   Trainer's License #

_____   _____

Date   State Licensed

FIGURE C-15

Process Validation Record

TPN Preparation

Student Name: _____   Date: _____

PROCEDURE	Yes	No
Followed proper hand-washing procedure and technique		
Wore appropriate apparel		
Followed proper procedure and technique in cleaning the hood		
Performed all necessary calculations correctly, prior to drug preparation		
Brought the correct drugs and concentrations into the hood for preparation		
Brought the correct supplies into the hood prior to preparation		
Inspected all products for particulate matter/contamination prior to use		
Withdrew electrolytes from vial according to proper procedures		
Added electrolytes to bottle of dextrose utilizing the vacuum inside the container		
Did not combine calcium- and phosphate-containing electrolytes inside the dextrose container		
Combined dextrose and amino acid solutions by adding to TPN bag		
Added phosphate-containing electrolytes to TPN bag after dextrose, amino acid, and other electrolytes had been added		
Visually inspected TPN for particulate contamination		
Added lipids last, if order called for a 3 in 1		
Properly mixed contents of TPN container		
Properly sealed additive port of TPN container		
Properly disconnected tubing from TPN bag and removed all air		
Properly sealed TPN bag where base solution was added		
Did not contaminate the needle or syringe during preparation		
Did not contaminate the hood		
Did not block airflow from HEPA filter or air intake grills at any time		
Did not utilize outer 6 in. of the hood opening		
Properly discarded all waste, including sharps		

By signing below, I certify that the student has demonstrated 100% competency at the above task.

_____   _____
Trainer Name (printed)   Trainer Signature

FIGURE C-16

Process Validation Record

Ampule Preparation—Hazardous Drugs

Student Name: _____ Date: _____

PROCEDURE	Yes	No
Followed proper hand-washing procedure and technique		
Wore appropriate apparel		
Followed proper procedure and technique in cleaning the hood		
Knew location of spill kit		
Knew location of eye wash station		
Performed all necessary calculations correctly prior to drug preparation		
Placed prep mat/paper drape correctly prior to drug preparation		
Brought the correct drugs and concentrations into the hood for preparation		
Brought the correct supplies into the hood prior to preparation		
Inspected all products for particulate matter/contamination prior to use		
Cleared ampule neck of fluid before breaking		
Cleaned ampule neck correctly before breaking		
Wrapped ampule neck correctly before breaking		
Broke ampule correctly		
Attached filter device to syringe correctly		
Drew up ampule correctly, without spilling contents		
Removed filter needle and replaced it with new needle prior to injecting into final container		
Drew up the correct amount of drug and checked measurement prior to injecting into container		
Cleaned additive port on final container prior to injecting drug		
Did not core or puncture side of additive port when adding drug to the final container		
Properly mixed contents of container and inspected for incompatibilities or particulate matter		
Placed IV container in a zip-lock bag before removal from the hood		
Used any and all appropriate hazardous labeling (for product and waste)		
Properly sealed additive port of container		
Did not contaminate the needle or syringe during preparation		
Did not contaminate the hood		
Did not block airflow from HEPA filter or air intake grills at any time		
Did not utilize outer 6 in. of the hood opening		
Properly discarded all waste, including sharps		

By signing below, I certify that the student has demonstrated 100% competency at the above task.

_____
Trainer Name (printed)

_____
Trainer Signature

_____   _____
Trainer Daytime Phone   Trainer's License #

_____   _____
Date   State Licensed

FIGURE C-17   Copyright © NPTA. All rights reserved.

Process Validation Record

Vial Preparation—Hazardous Drugs

Student Name: _____   Date: _____

PROCEDURE	Yes	No
Followed proper hand-washing procedure and technique		
Wore appropriate apparel		
Followed proper procedure and technique in cleaning the hood		
Knew location of spill kit		
Knew location of eye wash station		
Performed all necessary calculations correctly prior to drug preparation		
Placed prep-mat/paper drape correctly prior to drug preparation		
Brought the correct drugs and concentrations into the hood for preparation		
Brought the correct supplies into the hood prior to preparation		
Inspected all products for particulate matter/contamination prior to use		
Removed dust covers and cleaned rubber diaphragms correctly		
Inserted needle correctly to prevent coring		
Used proper milking technique or venting device and didn't aspirate at any time		
Did not remove needle from vial until all air bubbles were removed and amount verified		
Removed air bubbles correctly and did not spill any liquid		
Withdrew needle correctly from vial to prevent spilling or aspiration		
Cleaned additive port on final container prior to injecting drug		
Did not core or puncture side of additive port when adding drug to the final container		
Properly mixed contents of container and inspected for incompatibilities or particulate matter		
Properly sealed additive port of container		
Placed IV container in a zip-lock bag before removal from the hood		
Used any and all appropriate hazardous labeling (for product and waste)		
Did not contaminate the needle or syringe during preparation		
Did not contaminate the hood		
Did not block airflow from HEPA filter or air intake grills at any time		
Did not utilize outer 6 in. of the hood opening		
Properly discarded all waste, including sharps		

By signing below, I certify that the student has demonstrated 100% competency at the above task.

_____

Trainer Name (printed)

_____

Trainer Signature

_____   _____

Trainer Daytime Phone   Trainer's License #

_____   _____

Date   State Licensed

FIGURE C-18

Process Validation Record

Sterile Ophthalmic Solution Preparation

Student Name: _____   Date: _____

PROCEDURE	Yes	No
Used horizontal airflow hood or other form of Class 100 sterile environment		
All containers, closures, droppers, and equipment were sterile		
Selected appropriate container and closure		
Selected appropriate preservative/buffer if needed		
Used appropriate filtration device		
Used proper aseptic technique		
Properly closed and sealed product before removal		
Used appropriate autoclave procedures if needed		
Did not remove hands from hood at any time during preparation		
Brought correct supplies and equipment to the hood		
Did not block the HEPA filter		
Placed appropriate labels on the final product		
Product was stored appropriately, or dispensed immediately		

By signing below, I certify that the student has demonstrated 100% competency at the above task.

_____
Trainer Name (printed)

_____
Trainer Signature

_____
Trainer Daytime Phone   Trainer's License # _____

_____
Date   State Licensed _____

FIGURE C-19

Process Validation Record

Sterile Product Label Preparation

Student Name: _____   Date: _____

PROCEDURE	Yes	No
Label followed the appropriate format, approved by the institution		
Label contained the name and amount of all solutions		
Label contained the name and amount of all additives		
Label contained name and identification/room number of the patient		
Label contained rate of administration, if applicable		
Label contained proper storage information		
Label contained date and time for administration		
Label contained an expiration date		
Label contained identification of the preparer and pharmacist in charge		
Label was properly affixed		
Label did not contain any errors or corrections		
Performed appropriate calculations as required to prepare the label		
Accurately transcribed information on the label from the physician's order		

By signing below, I certify that the student has demonstrated 100% competency at the above task.

_____

Trainer Name (printed)

_____

Trainer Signature

_____   _____

Trainer Daytime Phone   Trainer's License #

_____   _____

Date   State Licensed

FIGURE C-20

Appendix D
Instructions for Left-Handed Personnel

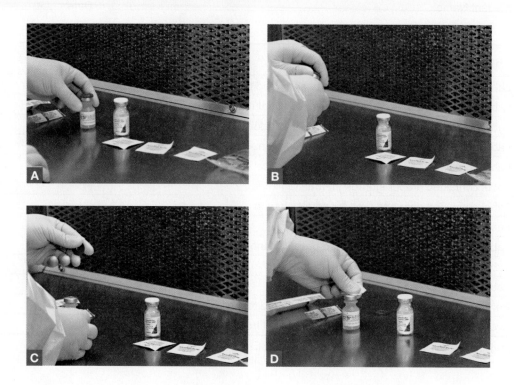

FIGURE D-1 Opening a vial (left hand)

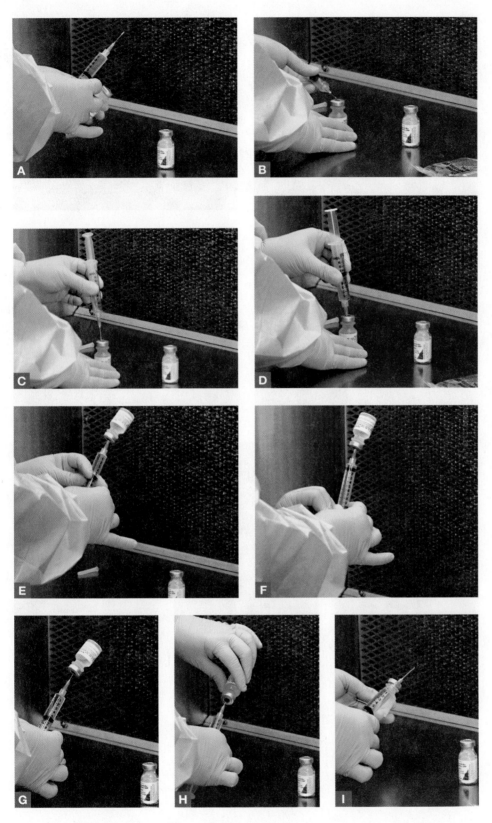

FIGURE D-2 Straight draw (left hand)

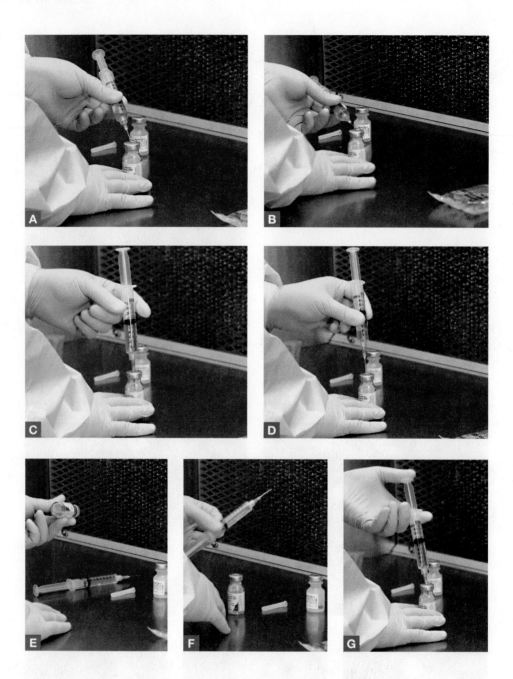

FIGURE D-3 Reconstitution of a lyophilized powder (left hand)

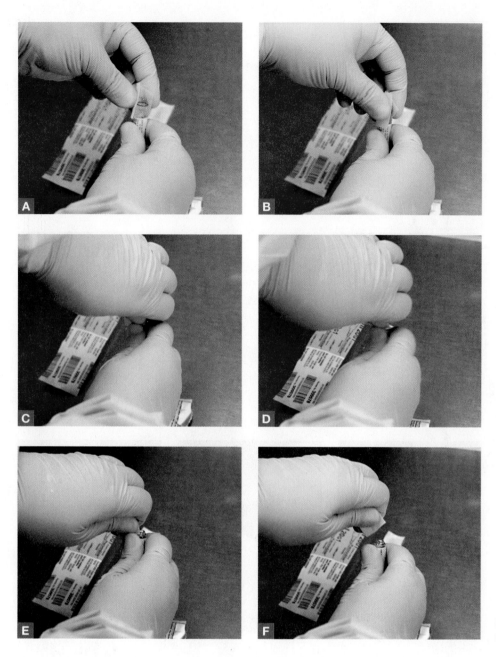

FIGURE D-4 Opening/breaking an ampule (left hand)

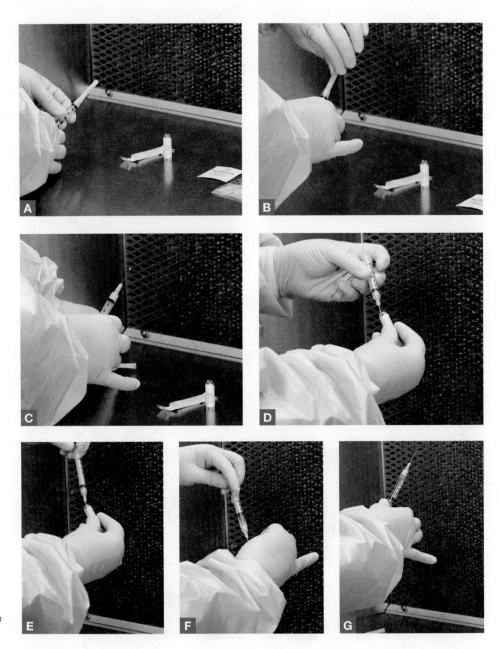

FIGURE D-5 Withdrawing fluid from an ampule (left hand)

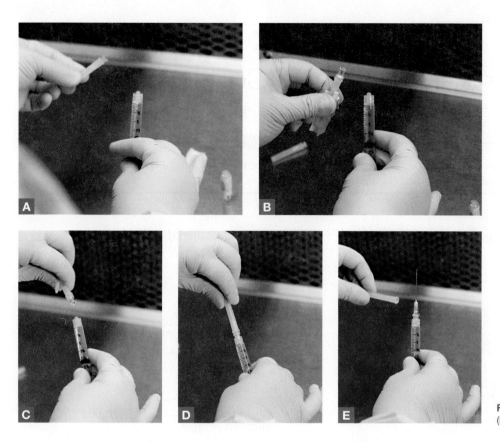

FIGURE D-6 Changing a needle (left hand)

Appendix E
Institutional Intravenous Certification Test

INFORMATION

Instructors can find the answers in the Instructor's Resource Manual files or by contacting the National Pharmacy Technician Association for online access.

---

1. The fast parenteral route of administration is _____.
   a. IM
   b. SQ
   c. ID
   d. IV

2. Which of the following materials should not be found in an anteroom?
   a. shoe covers
   b. lint-free towels
   c. cardboard boxes
   d. latex gloves

3. Rx: Penicillin G potassium 500,000 units IVPB q6h.

   After reconstitution, the vial concentration is 5,000,000 units/20 mL. How many milliliters of penicillin should be drawn up for each IVPB?
   a. 0.5 mL
   b. 1 mL
   c. 2 mL
   d. 4 mL

4. The precipitation of two drugs when added together indicates a _____ incompatibility.
   a. chemical
   b. therapeutic
   c. physical
   d. physiologic

5. IVPB is also known as _____.
   a. LVP
   b. LVIV
   c. SVP
   d. TPN

6. All PPE should be made of disposable, nonshedding low-permeability material.
   a. true
   b. false

7. An injection directly into the eye is _____.
   a. intraophthalmic
   b. intraotic
   c. intrapleural
   d. intraocular

8. Sterile 70% isopropyl alcohol is the only substance used to clean PECs.
   a. true
   b. false

9. In a TPN, _____ provide(s) patients with a source of protein.
   a. dextrose
   b. amino acids
   c. lipids
   d. sterile water

10. Rx: Heparin 20,000 units in D5W 1000 mL.
    Drug available: Heparin 10,000 units/mL 2 mL sdv.
    How much heparin would be injected into the D5W 1000-mL bag?
    a. 1 mL
    b. 2 mL
    c. 4 mL
    d. 8 mL

11. An IVP is injected or infused using a syringe.
    a. true
    b. false

12. When two drugs are added together causing a molecular change in one or both of the drugs, this is called a _____ incompatibility.
    a. chemical
    b. therapeutic
    c. physical
    d. physiologic

13. PPE can be worn outside the compounding area as long as it is not worn outdoors.
    a. true
    b. false

14. An infusion given via a central access catheter can be injected into _____.
    a. the jugular vein
    b. the subclavian vein
    c. the veins of arm
    d. the superior vena cava vein
    e. a, b, or d

15. Slip-tip syringes are the best choice for chemotherapy preparation.
    a. true
    b. false

16. A 1-g antibiotic vial states "Reconstitute with 4.8 mL of sterile water for a final volume of 5 mL." What is the powder volume in the vial?
    a. 5 mL
    b. 0.6 mL
    c. 0.2 mL
    d. 4.8 mL

17. When two or more drugs are given together or within a short period of each other resulting in the decreased effect of one or both of the drugs, this result is best described as a _____ incompatibility.
    a. chemical
    b. therapeutic
    c. physical
    d. physiologic

18. Gloves do not have to be disinfected as long as the technician properly performs aseptic hand washing.
    a. true
    b. false

19. PCA is the abbreviation for patient-concentrated analgesics.
    a. true
    b. false

20. Vitamin B_{12} is the abbreviation for _____.
    a. thiamine
    b. pyridoxine
    c. ascorbic acid
    d. cyanocobalamin

21. In a TPN, _____ provide(s) patients with a source of carbohydrates.
    a. dextrose
    b. amino acids
    c. lipids
    d. sterile water

22. The anteroom must be maintained as an _____ or better environment.
    a. ISO 5
    b. ISO 6

    c. ISO 7
    d. ISO 8

23. A 1 g antibiotic vial states "Reconstitute with 4.8 mL of sterile water for a final volume of 5 mL." What is the drug concentration in the vial?
    a. 1 g/4.8 mL
    b. 100 mg/mL
    c. 1000 mg/mL
    d. 200 mg/mL

24. A pH level of 3 is considered _____.
    a. basic
    b. acidic
    c. alkaline
    d. either a or c

25. USP 797 allows for the use of antimicrobial or nonantimicrobial soap for hand washing.
    a. true
    b. false

26. An infusion given at a continuous rate over a long period of time is best described as _____.
    a. a bolus
    b. TPN
    c. a continuous infusion
    d. an intravenous piggyback

27. Filter needles should always be used when withdrawing medication from a (an) _____.
    a. single-dose vial
    b. multiple-dose vial
    c. ampule
    d. sterile vial

28. How much 4-mEq/mL NaCl must be drawn up for a 42-mEq dose?
    a. 4.2 mL
    b. 10 mL
    c. 10.5 mL
    d. 12.6 mL

29. Low-risk compounded sterile products must be prepared in an _____ environment.
    a. ISO 4
    b. ISO 5
    c. ISO 7
    d. ISO 8

30. Counters, work surfaces, and floors must be cleaned and disinfected _____.
    a. every 30 min
    b. every 6 hr
    c. daily
    d. monthly

31. In a TPN, _____ provide(s) patients with a source of fats.
    a. dextrose
    b. amino acids
    c. lipids
    d. sterile water

32. A pH level of 9.6 is considered _____.
    a. basic
    b. acidic
    c. alkaline
    d. either a or c

33. Paper waste from syringes should always be placed in the DCA to prevent contamination.
    a. true
    b. false

34. Infusions given via the following route(s) must not contain preservatives:
    a. intracardiac
    b. epidural
    c. intrathecal
    d. intrapleural
    e. both b and c

35. Common TPN bags range in size from 500 mL to _____.
    a. 1000 mL
    b. 4000 mL
    c. 5000 mL
    d. 6000 mL

36. The part of the needle that attaches to the syringe is called the _____.
    a. bevel
    b. shaft
    c. hub
    d. plunger

37. What is the IV flow rate of 2000 mL infused over 8 hr?
    a. 125 mL/hr
    b. 200 mL/hr
    c. 250 mL/hr
    d. 500 mL/hr

38. Which of the following is NOT one of the "Seven Rights" of medication administration?
    a. right medication
    b. right ROA
    c. right doctor
    d. right dose

39. A _____ incompatibility can most likely be visibly observed.
    a. chemical
    b. physical

    c. therapeutic
    d. physiologic

40. The standard size needles used by pharmacy when compounding sterile products is _____.
    a. 27 G
    b. 14 G
    c. 13 G
    d. 18 G

41. Which of the following is used to prevent and treat hypovolemic shock?
    a. IVIG
    b. IGG
    c. PPF
    d. factor VIII

42. In a TPN, _____ is (are) used to adjust the volume of the infusion.
    a. dextrose
    b. amino acids
    c. lipids
    d. sterile water

43. Skin tests are commonly given via the _____ route.
    a. IV
    b. IM
    c. ID
    d. SQ

44. Which of the following parts of the syringe holds and measures the medication?
    a. tip
    b. plunger
    c. flange
    d. barrel

45. How long will a 500 mL IV bag last if it is infused at a rate of 25 mL/hr?
    a. 1 hr
    b. 5 hr
    c. 10 hr
    d. 20 hr

46. A solution with a higher concentration of solute as compared to blood is considered _____.
    a. isotonic
    b. hypotonic
    c. hypertonic

47. USP 797 suggests that the BUD of a MDV is _____ days unless otherwise noted by the vial's manufacturer.
    a. 10
    b. 20

c. 28

d. 30

48. Ophthalmic products must remain sterile.

    a. true

    b. false

49. USP 797 provides accreditation to hospital pharmacies after they adhere to strict guidelines and inspections.

    a. true

    b. false

50. Each gram of _____ provides 3.45 calories.

    a. dextrose

    b. amino acids

    c. lipids

    d. sterile water

51. Low-molecular-weight heparin is commonly given via the _____ route.

    a. IV

    b. IM

    c. ID

    d. SQ

52. High-risk compounded sterile products are those exposed for more than 1 hr to an environment worse than _____.

    a. ISO 4

    b. ISO 5

    c. ISO 7

    d. ISO 8

53. PECs must maintain an _____ or better environment.

    a. ISO 5

    b. ISO 6

    c. ISO 7

    d. ISO 8

54. Rx: NS at 100 mL/hr.

    IV set drop rate: 10 gtt/mL.

    What is the drip rate for this IV?

    a. 10 gtt/min

    b. 11 gtt/min

    c. 16 gtt/min

    d. 17 gtt/min

55. Which of the following is used to prevent and control bleeding?

    a. IVIG

    b. IGG

    c. PPF

    d. factor VIII

56. A solution with the same concentration of solute as compared to blood is considered _____.

    a. isotonic

    b. hypotonic

    c. hypertonic

57. Which of the following is the last additive injected into a TPN bag?

    a. sodium chloride

    b. calcium chloride

    c. potassium chloride

    d. multiple-vitamin injection

58. Any syringe used in the preparation of chemotherapy medications should not be filled more than _____ full of drug.

    a. 20%

    b. 25%

    c. 50%

    d. 75%

59. Ampules should always be broken towards the HEPA filter of a PEC.

    a. true

    b. false

60. Drugs used to compound epidurals must be preservative free.

    a. true

    b. false

61. An initial dose of a drug that is used to achieve a desired drug level is best described as _____.

    a. a loading dose

    b. a bolus

    c. a continuous infusion

    d. an intravenous piggyback

    e. both a and b

62. Which of the following are considered PECs?

    a. LAFW

    b. BSC

    c. CAI

    d. CACI

    e. all of the above

63. How many grams of dextrose are contained in 2 L of D5W?

    a. 5

    b. 10

    c. 50

    d. 100

64. A solution with a lower concentration of solute as compared to blood is considered _____.

    a. isotonic

    b. hypotonic

    c. hypertonic

65. The direction of airflow in a BSC is _____.
    a. vertical from the bottom
    b. horizontal from the top
    c. vertical from the top
    d. horizontal from the back

66. Which of the following helps to build, repair, and maintain body tissues?
    a. dextrose
    b. amino acids
    c. lipids
    d. sterile water

67. A pharmacy technician should never use the same needle that is used to withdraw liquid from an ampule to inject that liquid into an IV bag.
    a. true
    b. false

68. Delivery of a secondary IV solution into an existing IV line is best described as _____.
    a. intermittent infusion
    b. continuous infusion
    c. intravenous piggyback
    d. a bolus

69. Which of the following is not a glovebox isolator?
    a. CAI
    b. CACI
    c. BSC
    d. LAFW
    e. both c and d

70. If you use 10 g of drug to prepare 1 L of an IV solution, what is the percentage strength of the final product?
    a. 0.1%
    b. 1%
    c. 10%
    d. 15%

71. An infusion of a hypertonic solution would cause the surrounding blood cells to _____.
    a. expand
    b. shrink
    c. stay the same
    d. do none of the above

72. All needles and syringes used in the preparation of chemotherapy must be disposed of in a _____.
    a. red sharps container
    b. hazardous soft waste container
    c. hazardous/chemotherapy sharps container
    d. regular trash can

73. Which of the following electrolytes contributes to proper nerve and muscle function?
    a. sodium
    b. calcium
    c. potassium
    d. phosphate

74. According to USP 797, which of the following is completed first when donning PPE?
    a. face/eye masks
    b. shoe covers
    c. aseptically wash hands
    d. head and facial hair covers

75. An injection directly into the peritoneal cavity or into an abdominal organ such as the kidney, liver, or bladder is best described as the _____ route.
    a. intraperitoneal
    b. intrapleural
    c. intracardiac
    d. intramuscular

76. The compounding aseptic isolator uses positive pressure to protect personnel and CSPs.
    a. true
    b. false

77. You need to prepare 1 L of D40W using both D70W and D5W. How much D70W is needed?
    a. 236.4 mL
    b. 461.5 mL
    c. 538.5 mL
    d. 763.6 mL

78. An infusion of a hypotonic solution would cause the surrounding blood cells to _____.
    a. expand
    b. shrink
    c. stay the same
    d. do none of the above

79. When preparing chemotherapy medications, the needles should not be recapped before disposal.
    a. true
    b. false

80. According to USP 797, which of the following is completed last when donning PPE?
    a. face/eye masks
    b. shoe covers
    c. aseptically wash hands
    d. gloves

81. An injection directly into the heart is best described as being by the _____ route.
    a. intraperitoneal
    b. intrapleural

c. intracardiac

d. intramuscular

82. Glovebox isolators can be used to compound sterile products when the pharmacy does not have a clean room.

   a. true

   b. false

83. You need to prepare 1 L of D40W using both D70W and D5W. How much D5W do you need?

   a. 236.4 mL

   b. 461.5 mL

   c. 538.5 mL

   d. 763.6 mL

84. According to USP 797, which of the following is first when removing PPE?

   a. face/eye masks

   b. shoe covers

   c. gown

   d. gloves

85. Which of the following electrolytes determines total body water?

   a. sodium

   b. calcium

   c. potassium

   d. phosphate

86. A small chemotherapy spill is anything less than _____.

   a. 1 mL

   b. 3 mL

   c. 5 mL

   d. 10 mL

87. The direction of airflow of a (an) _____ is horizontal from back to front.

   a. BSC

   b. LAFW

   c. CAI

   d. PEC

88. B_6 is the abbreviation for _____.

   a. thiamine

   b. cyanocobalamin

   c. pyridoxine

   d. ascorbic acid

89. Rx: Zinacef 750 mg IVPB in D5W 50 mL, infuse over 30 min q12h.

   The 1.5-g cefuroxime vial states that if you "reconstitute with 7.5 mL the resulting final volume of the vial is 10 mL."

   If you want to change the concentration, how much diluent should you add to obtain a vial concentration of 1.5 g/20mL?

   a. 7.5 mL

   b. 10 mL

   c. 15 mL

   d. 20 mL

90. USP requires ceilings and walls to be cleaned and disinfected _____.

   a. every 30 min

   b. every 6 hr

   c. daily

   d. monthly

91. The _____ of a solution is the number of osmoles of solute per liter of solution.

   a. molality

   b. molarity

   c. osmolality

   d. osmolarity

92. USP 797 does not recommend the use of which of the following during hand washing?

   a. lint-free towels

   b. antimicrobial soap

   c. paper towels

   d. nontouch electric hand dryers

93. TPN with a dextrose concentration above 10% must be given via a _____ line.

   a. central

   b. peripheral

94. USP requires that PECs be cleaned and disinfected every _____ min during times of continuous compounding of sterile products.

   a. 15

   b. 30

   c. 45

   d. 60

95. When the pharmacy dispenses a chemotherapy infusion with an IV set, the technician primes the IV set after he or she adds the chemotherapy to the IV bag.

   a. true

   b. false

96. When giving IM volumes greater than 3 mL, the dose should be divided into two injections.

   a. true

   b. false

97. Rx: Zinacef 750 mg IVPB in D5W 50 mL, infuse over 30 min q12h.

   The 1.5-g cefuroxime vial states that if you "reconstitute with 7.5 mL the resulting final volume of the vial is 10 mL." If the vial is diluted to 1.5 g/20mL, how much drug should you draw up for one dose?

   a. 7.5 mL

   b. 10 mL

c. 15 mL

d. 20 mL

98. When beginning a TPN infusion, the infusion must be tapered up over several hours to the correct rate.

a. true

b. false

99. To increase accuracy, the volume being measured in a syringe must be at least _____ of the maximum capacity of the syringe.

a. 10%

b. 20%

c. 25%

d. 75%

100. When cleaning a LAFW, the technician should always start with the work surface.

a. true

b. false

101. A (an) _____ is used to clean peripheral access lines and aids in preventing blood coagulation.

a. low-molecular-weight-heparin flush

b. insulin flush

c. normal saline flush

d. heparin-lock flush

102. Rx: Zinacef 750 mg IVPB in D5W 50 mL, infuse over 30 min q12h.

The 1.5-g cefuroxime vial states that if you "reconstitute with 7.5 mL the resulting final volume of the vial is 10 mL." How many doses are available in one 1.5-g vial?

a. one

b. two

c. three

d. four

103. What is used on the surface of a BSC when preparing chemotherapy infusions?

a. sticky mat

b. lint-free towels

c. chemotherapy mat

d. paper towels

104. The bevel of a needle is the pointed end of the needle.

a. true

b. false

105. Blood has an approximate pH level of _____.

a. 6.7

b. 7.0

c. 7.4

d. 7.6

106. Syringe tip caps should always be removed prior to placing the syringe into the PEC.

a. true

b. false

107. An injection of 10 mL or less directly from a syringe into the vein is best described as _____.

a. an intermittent infusion

b. IVP

c. IVPB

d. a bolus

108. ISO 5 is equivalent to a Class 100 environment.

a. true

b. false

109. Which of the following would be the first additive to a TPN?

a. calcium

b. potassium

c. phosphate

d. sodium

110. Rx: Zinacef 750 mg IVPB in D5W 50 mL, infuse over 30 min q12h.

The 1.5-g cefuroxime vial states that if you "reconstitute with 7.5 mL the resulting final volume of the vial is 10 mL." How many vials are needed to prepare a 7-day supply?

a. two

b. four

c. six

d. seven

Index

A

Abbott's Nitrimix Macro, 95
Abbreviations
  chemical, 6–7
  infusion fluid, 81
  intravenous solution, 6
  sterile product, 7–8
Acid, 134
Acidic, 54, 57
Acidic solutions, 54, 55
Additive, 4, 134
Administration routes. See Routes of
  administration
Admixture, 4, 134
Advantage bags, 25
Aerosolization, 4, 111, 115, 134
Aerosols, 112
Air bubbles, in syringes, 67
Air environments, 13–14
Albumin, 84–85, 134
Alcohol
  benzyl, 83
  isopropyl, 17, 61, 63
  swabbing with, 63, 73
Alcohol pads, 21, 63
Alkaline, 54, 57, 134
Alkaline solutions, 54, 55
Alligations, 42–46
Alphanate (Factor VIII), 85–86
American Society of Health-System
  Pharmacists (ASHP), 12, 56, 63
  on cytotoxic agents, 114–115
  on quality assurance, 120–126
  on small spills, 114
Amino acids, 90, 91, 134
Ampule Preparation Form, 153–154
Ampule Preparation–Hazardous Drugs
  Form, 156
Ampules
  explanation of, 4, 23, 69, 134
  forms for preparation of, 153–154, 156
  left-handed technicians using,
    163, 164
  removing fluid from, 71–72
  use of, 69–71
Analgesia, patient-controlled, 83
Ante area, 134
Anteroom, 14, 27
Antibacterial, 135
Antibiotic, 134
Anticoagulant, 134
Antimicrobial, 134
Antineoplastics, 101, 115, 134. See also
  Cytotoxic agents
Asepsis, 134
Aseptic, 2, 134
Aseptic calculations
  alligations and, 42–46
  dilute, powder and final volume of
    reconstituted power vials and, 33–35
  dilution technique and, 48

electrolytes added to total parenteral
  nutrition preparations and, 46–48
intravenous additive dosage and, 31–33
intravenous drip rates and, 37–39
intravenous flow rates and, 36–37
intravenous frequency or schedule and, 37
milliequivalents and, 36
percentage concentrations and, 39–42
Aseptic Hand Washing Technique Form, 150
Aseptic technique
  air bubble removal and, 67
  alcohol swabbing and, 63, 73
  ampule use and, 69–72
  ASHP guidelines for, 122–124, 126
  for chemotherapy medications, 110, 115
  for compounding, 2
  explanation of, 4, 60, 75, 134
  forms for, 140–150
  hand washing and, 61, 62, 150
  manipulation and, 63, 67–72
  needle use and, 64
  proper dress and, 61
  standards of practice, 74–77
  sterile dosage form preparation and,
    72–73
  syringe use and, 63–64
  for total parenteral nutrition
    preparation, 90
  transfer needle use and, 67–69
  vial use and, 64–67
Aseptic Technique Training Log, 140–149
Attire
  for aseptic technique, 61
  ASHP guidelines for, 122, 124, 126
  for compounding chemotherapy
    medications, 109
  personal protection equipment, 19–20
Autoclave, 134
Automated devices, for TPN preparation,
  95–96
Automix 3 + 3 compounder, 95
Auxiliary labels, 26
Avogadro's number, 57

B

B. Braun's Pinnacle compounder, 95
Bacteria, 17
Bacteriocidal, 4, 134
Bacteriostatic, 5, 134
Barrel, syringe, 23, 134
Bases, 54
Batch preparation, 134
Beard cover, 20
Benzyl alcohol, 83
Bevel, 21, 134
Bevel tip, 21
Beyond-use date (BUD), 134
Biological safety cabinets (BSCs)
  characteristics of, 105
  chemotherapy medications compounded in,
    102, 105–108

cleaning and decontaminating, 106–108
  explanation of, 15, 16, 102, 115, 134
  hood preparation for, 106
  proper use of, 106
  shutting down, 108
Blood, human, pH scale of, 54
Bolus, 5, 134
Brand-name intravenous medications,
  138–139
Buffer area, 14, 15, 134

C

Calcium, 91
Calories, for total parenteral nutrition, 90
Cancer
  explanation of, 99
  types of, 110
  viruses linked to, 110
Carbohydrates, 90
Carcinogenic, 115, 134
Carmel Pharma, Inc., 112
Centers for Disease Control and Prevention
  (CDC), 120
Central line, 4, 5, 93, 96, 134
Certification, national pharmacy technician, 27
Chemical abbreviations, 6–7
Chemical incompatibility, 55
Chemo pin, 134
Chemotherapy
  explanation of, 99, 115, 134
  uses for, 100
Chemotherapy mat (chemo mat), 102, 112,
  115, 134
Chemotherapy medications
  ASHP guidelines for handling, 114–115
  attire when working with, 109
  biological safety cabinet for
    compounding, 16
  cautions for working with, 115
  disposal of, 113
  handling spills of, 113–114
  method to compound, 84, 102, 105–108
  orders for, 102–104
  procedures for handling, 111–112
  training to mix, 108–109
  withdrawing, 110–111
Chemotherapy spill kits, 113, 114
Chloride, 91
Clean air space
  explanation of, 14–15
  opening syringe packages in, 63
Cleaning procedure, for PECs, 17–19
Clean rooms
  explanation of, 11, 13, 132, 134
  standards for, 124
  supplies in or near, 19
  USP 797 regulations for, 14
Clinitec, 95
Closed-system aseptic transfer, 121, 132, 134
Closed-system transfer device, 112
Compatibility, 5, 55–56, 135

Compounded sterile products (CSPs)
    guidelines for patients treated with, 12
    hazardous, 17
    risk levels for, 127–129
Compounding. *See also* Sterile compounding
    explanation of, 1, 121, 132, 135
    hazardous, 16
    supplies for, 21–23
Compounding areas
    cleaning and disinfecting, 129–130
    explanation of, 11
Compounding aseptic containment isolator
    (CACI), 16, 17
Compounding aseptic isolator (CAI),
    15–17
Contamination, 5, 135
Continuous infusion, 4, 5, 8, 135
Controlled areas, 122, 132, 134
Coring, 5, 53, 57, 135
Corrective action, 123, 132, 135
Critical area, 132, 135
Critical site, 5
Cytotoxic, 116, 135
Cytotoxic agents
    ASHP guidelines for handling,
        114–115
    attire when working with, 109
    biological safety cabinet for
        compounding, 16
    cautions for working with, 115
    compounding of, 84, 100
    disposal of, 113
    handling spills of, 113–114
    list of common, 101
    orders for, 102–104
    procedures for handling, 111–112
    training to mix, 108–109
    withdrawing, 110–111

D
Dark bags, 26
Decompensate, 135
Depth filters, 24
Desiccation, 27, 135
Dextrose, 54, 90
Diluent
    explanation of, 5, 135
    volume of, 33–35
Dilutions
    for neonates and pediatric patients, 83
    technique for, 48
Disinfectant, 135
Dispensing pins, 25, 26
Documentation, 123, 125, 126, 131
Dressings (garb)
    for aseptic technique, 61
    ASHP guidelines for, 122, 124, 126
    for compounding chemotherapy
        medications, 109
    personal protection equipment, 19–20
Drip rates
    explanation of, 36
    intravenous, 37–39
Drips, 82

E
Electrolytes
    explanation of, 47, 135
    in total parenteral nutrition preparations,
        46–48, 90, 91
Empty evacuated containers (EECs), 24
End-product evaluations, 123, 125, 126, 131

Enteral, 135
Environmental control, 13–14
Environmental sampling tests, 129
Enzymes, 135
Epidurals (EP), 3, 83, 135
Expiration dates, 123, 125, 126
Extravasation, 5

F
Factor IX (Konyne), 86
Factor VIII (Alphanate), 85–86
Filters
    depth, 24
    explanation of, 23–24
    HEPA, 16, 71, 73, 102, 105, 135
    inline, 24, 95
    membrane, 5
Fluid maintenance, for total parenteral
    nutrition, 90
Foil port covers, 26
Food and Drug Administration (FDA), 120
Fortaz, 80

G
Garb. *See* Dressings (garb)
Gastrointestinal tract, method to bypass, 2
Gauge, needle, 21, 22
Generic intravenous medications, 137–138
Gentamicin, 84
Gentamicin irrigation solution, 84
Germicidal, 17, 27, 135
Glovebox isolator, 16–17
Gloves, 19, 20, 61, 113–115
Good *Manufacturing Practices* (Food and
    Drug Administration), 120
Googles, 113, 115
Gowns, 20, 113, 115
Gravity filling, 135
*Guidelines on Quality Assurance for
    Pharmacy-Prepared Sterile Products*
    (American Society of Health-System
    Pharmacists), 120

H
Hair cover, 19, 20
Handbook of Injectable Drugs (Trissel), 56
Hand washing, 61, 62, 150
Hazardous materials
    ampule preparation form for, 156
    compounded sterile products as, 17
    method to compound, 16, 17
    vial preparation forms for, 157
    yellow disposal containers for, 113,
        116, 136
Heparin
    explanation of, 135
    flushing peripheral lines with, 4
    preparation precautions for, 32–33
Heparin-lock flush, 4
High-efficiency particulate air (HEPA) filters,
    16, 71, 73, 102, 105, 135
High-risk-level compounded sterile products,
    128–129
Horizontal Laminar Airflow Hood
    Form, 151
Horizontal laminar airflow hood
    (LAFW), 16
Hub, 21, 135
Hyperglycemia, 93, 96, 135
Hypertonic solutions, 56, 135
Hypoglycemia, 93, 96, 135
Hypotonic solutions, 56, 135

I
Immunocompromised, 61, 76, 135
Immunoglobulin (IgG), 85
Incompatibilities, 55–56
Infection, 2. *See also* Sepsis
Infiltration, 5
Infusion, 5, 135
Infusion fluid abbreviations, 81
Injectable routes of administration, 2
Inline filters, 24, 95
Institutional Intravenous Certification Test,
    166–172
Intermittent infusion, 5
International Organization for
    Standardization (ISO), categories for air
    environments, 13–14
International System of Units (SI System), 57
Intra-arterial (IA) injection, 3
Intracardiac (IC) injection, 3
Intradermal (ID) injection, 2
Intramuscular (IM) injection, 2, 135
Intraocular injection, 3
Intraperitoneal injection, 3
Intrapleural injection, 3
Intrathecal (IT) injection, 3, 135
Intravenous additive dosage, 31–33
Intravenous (IV) bags
    explanation of, 80
    large-volume intravenous and large-volume
        parenteral, 81
    piggyback, 80–81
Intravenous (IV) drip rate
    calculation of, 37–39
    explanation of, 37
Intravenous (IV) flow rates, 36–37
Intravenous (IV) frequency, 37
Intravenous (IV) infusions
    administration of, 3–4
    explanation of, 4
    preparation of, 1
Intravenous (IV) injection
    explanation of, 2–3, 135
    historical background of, 1
Intravenous (IV) lines, 4
Intravenous (IV) solution abbreviations, 6
Intravenous (IV) tubing, 24
Intravenous medications
    brand name, 138–139
    generic, 137–138
Intravenous piggybacks (ivpbs)
    explanation of, 5, 25, 80, 87, 135
    preparation of, 80–81
    transfer needles for, 67
Intravenous push (IVP)
    explanation of, 4, 8, 135
    syringes for, 82
Irrigation, 84, 87, 135
Iso-osmotic, 135
Isopropyl alcohol (IPA)
    to disinfect hands, 61
    for hood cleaning, 17
    swabbing with, 63
Isotonic solutions, 56, 57, 135
IVA seals, 26

J
Joint Commission (formerly Joint Commission
    on Accreditation of Healthcare
    Organizations (JCAHO), 120

K
Konyne (Factor IX), 86

L

Labels
  auxiliary, 26
  function of, 123, 125, 126
  process validation record for sterile
    products, 159
  quality control and, 131
Laminar airflow hoods
  explanation of, 15–16, 135
  horizontal, 16, 151
  vertical, 152
Large-volume intravenous (LVIV) bags, 81
Large-volume parenterals (LVPs), 81
Left-handed technicians, 160–165
Lipids, 90
Loading dose, 5, 135
Logarithmic, 54
Low-risk-level compounded sterile products
  explanation of, 127–128
Luer lock syringe, 23, 63
Luer-to-Luer connectors, 25, 26
Lumen, 21
Lyophilized medication, 135

M

Magnesium, 91
Male adapters, 26
Malignant, 99, 116, 135
Masks, 19, 20
Media-fill test, 136
Medications
  chemotherapy, 16, 84, 102–115
  intravenous, 137–139
  lyophilized, 135
  oral, 1
  topical, 1
Medium-risk-level compounded sterile
    products, 128
Membrane filters, 5
Metathesis, 136
Micromix compounder, 95–96
Millequivalents (mEqs), 36, 47
Minerals, for total parenteral nutrition, 91
Minibags, 25
Molality, 57
Molarity, 57
Mole, 57
Multiple-dose vial (MDV)
  explanation of, 5, 64
  use of, 82–83

N

Narcotic, 136
National Pharmacy Technician Association
    (NPTA), national certification by, 27
Needles
  changed by left-handed technicians, 165
  gauge of, 21, 22
  length of, 21, 22
  parts of, 21
  transfer, 67–69
  types of, 64
Neonates
  dilutions for, 83
  explanation of, 96
Neosporin, 84
Nitrimix Macro (Abbot), 95
Nonsterile compounding, 1

O

Occupational Safety and Health
    Administration (OSHA), 113, 114

Ophthalmics, 86
Ophthalmic solutions, 86, 158
Osmolality, 56–57, 136
Osmolarity, 56–57, 136
Osmole, 57
Osmosis, 136

P

Parenteral, 5
Parenteral injection
  aseptic technique for, 4
  explanation of, 2, 8, 136
  routes of administration for, 2–3
Particulates, 13, 27, 54, 136
Pathogen, 5
Patient-controlled analgesia (PCA), 83
Pediatric patients, 83
Percentage concentrations
  calculation of, 39–42
  classification of, 39
Peripheral line
  explanation of, 3–5, 93, 96
  flushing of, 4
Personal protection equipment (PPE), 19–20, 61
Pharmacy technicians. *See also* Training
  instructions for left-handed, 160–165
  requirements and certification for, 27
  role in compounding sterile products, 8
  training for, 27, 108–109, 122, 124
PhaSeal, 112, 113
Phlebitis, 8, 136
Phosphate, 91
pH scale, 54–55
Physical incompatibility, 55
Piggyback (IVPB), 4, 8
Pinnacle compounder (B. Braun), 95
Plasma protein fraction (PPF), 85
Plunger, syringe, 23
Port adapters, 26
Positive pressure, 64, 136
Potassium, 91
Potassium chloride (KCl), 73, 80, 93
Powders, method to weigh, 33
Powder volume (PV), 34–35
Preservative, 5, 136
Primary engineering controls (PECs)
  biological safety cabinet and, 16
  explanation of, 14–16
  glovebox isolator and, 16–17
  hood cleaning and, 17–19
  horizontal laminar airflow hood
    and, 16
Primary tubing, 24
Process validation
  explanation of, 19, 123, 124, 126,
    130–132, 136
  forms for, 150–159
Process validation records
  Ampule Preparation, 153–154
  Ampule Preparation–Hazardous
    Drugs, 156
  Aseptic Hand Washing Technique, 150
  Horizontal Laminar Airflow Hood, 151
  Sterile Ophthalmic Solution Preparation,
    158
  Sterile Product Label Preparation, 159
  TPN Preparation, 155
  Vertical Laminar Airflow Hood, 152
  Vial Preparation – Hazardous Drugs, 157
Proteins, 84
Protocol, 96, 136
Pyrogen, 4, 5, 8, 136

Q

Quality assurance
  ASHP guidelines for, 121–126
  elements of, 119–120
  explanation of, 118, 119, 132, 136
  functions of, 119
  guidelines for, 120–121
  for levels of risk, 127–129
Quality control
  documentation and labeling for, 131
  explanation of, 118, 119, 132, 136
  USP 797 standards for, 126–131
Quality improvement, 119–120

R

Ratio proportion, 31–33
Reconstitute, 136
Reconstitution
  explanation of, 5, 64, 76
  by left-handed technicians, 162
  of powder vials, 33–35
Red sharps containers, 26
Renal failure, 136
Respirators, 115
Risk level 1, 121–123
Risk level 2, 123–125
Risk level 3, 125–126
Routes of administration
  intravenous, 3–4
  parenteral, 2–3

S

Saline, 4
Sanitation, 136
Scrubs, 20
Sepsis, 2, 8, 136
Shadowing, 105, 116, 136
Shaft, 21
Shoe covers, 19, 20
Single-dose vials (SDVs)
  explanation of, 5, 23, 27, 136
  use of, 64
Slip tip syringe, 23
Small-volume parenterals (SVPs), 80
Sodium, 91
Solute, 136
Solutions. *See also specific solutions*
  acidic, 54, 55
  alkaline, 54, 55
  hypertonic, 56
  hypotonic, 56
  isotonic, 56, 57
Specific gravity, 95, 96, 136
Stability, 56
Standard order, for total parenteral
    nutrition, 92
Sterile, 2
Sterile compounding. *See also* Compounding;
    USP 797 Guidebook to Pharmaceutical
    Compounding–Sterile Preparations
    (USP 797)
  clear air space for, 14–15
  explanation of, 1, 2, 5
  requirements for, 11, 31, 122–123
Sterile dosage forms, 72, 73
Sterile Ophthalmic Solution Preparation
    Form, 158
Sterile product certification courses, 27
Sterile Product Label Preparation Form, 159
Sterile product preparations
  albumin and, 84–85
  cytotoxic medications and, 84

Sterile product preparations (*continued*)
    factor IX and, 86
    factor VIII and, 85–86
    immunoglobulin and, 85
    intravenous bags and, 80–82
    irrigations and, 84
    multidose vials and, 64, 82–83
    for neonates and pediatric patients, 83
    ophthalmics and, 86
    patient-controlled analgesia and, 83
    plasma protein fraction and, 85
    proteins and, 84
    requirements for, 79
    syringes and, 82
    total parenteral nutrition and, 84
Sterile products
    abbreviations for, 7–8
    aseptic technique and, 8
    compatibility and stability and, 55–56
    high-risk-level compounded, 128–129
    low-risk-level compounded, 127–128
    medium-risk-level compounded, 128
    osmolality and osmolarity and, 56–57
    particulate matter and, 54
    pH, acids and bases and, 54–55
    preparation of, 53
    properties of, 53–57
    role of pharmacy technician in
        compounding, 8
    terminology for, 4–5
    tonicity and, 56
Sterile water, 90
Sterile water for injection (SWFI), 64
Sterility, 136
Sticky mats, 23, 136
Straight draw, by left-handed technicians, 161
Subcutaneous (SC, SQ, subq) injection,
    2, 136
Surgical antibiotic solution, 84
Syringe caps, 25, 26
Syringes
    explanation of, 21
    for intravenous push, 82
    locking mechanisms on, 63–64
    Luer lock, 23, 63
    methods to use, 63
    parts of, 21–23
    removal of air bubbles from, 67
    slip tip, 23
    variations in, 23, 63

T
*Technical Assistance Bulletin on Handling
    Cytotoxic and Hazardous Drugs*
    (American Society of Health-System
    Pharmacists), 114–115
Teratogenic, 101, 116, 136
Therapeutic incompatibility, 55
Tip, syringe, 21
Tonicity, 56
Topical medications, 1
Total parenteral nutrition (TPN)
    amino acids and, 91
    automated devices for, 95–96
    calories and carbohydrates and, 90
    components of, 90
    compounding of, 84, 93–95
    controversy over use of, 96
    electrolytes added to, 46–48
    electrolytes and minerals and, 91
    explanation of, 89
    fluid maintenance and, 90
    order for, 91–93
    preparation forms for, 155, 156
TPN Preparation Form, 155
Trace elements, 90
Training
    ASHP guidelines for, 122, 124, 125
    forms for, 140–159
    to mix chemotherapy products, 108–109
    sterile product certification courses, 27
Training and validation forms
    Ampule Preparation, 153–154
    Ampule Preparation – Hazardous
        Drugs, 156
    Aseptic Hand Washing Technique, 150
    Aseptic Technique Training Log, 140–149
    Horizontal Laminar Airflow Hood, 151
    Sterile Ophthalmic Solution
        Preparation, 158
    Sterile Product Label Preparation, 159
    TPN Preparation, 155
    Vertical Laminar Airflow Hood, 152
    Vial Preparation–Hazardous Drugs, 157
Transfer needles, 67–69
Trissel, L. A., 56

U
U.S. Pharmacopeia, USP 797 Guidebook to
    Pharmaceutical Compounding–Sterile
    Preparations (USP 797), 11–26, 121

USP 797 Guidebook to Pharmaceutical
    Compounding–Sterile Preparations
    (USP 797)
    clean air space, 14–15
    clean room, 13, 14
    compounding supplies, 21–23
    dressing (garb), 19–20, 61
    environmental sampling tests
        and, 129
    explanation of, 11–13, 27, 121
    facilities, 13–14
    miscellaneous equipment, 23–26
    primary engineering controls,
        15–19
    quality control and, 126–131
    standards of practice, 74–75
    syringes, 23

V
Vented tubing, 24
Vertical airflow hood, 16
Vertical Laminar Airflow Hood
    Form, 152
Viaflex bags, 25
Vial Preparation–Hazardous Drugs
    Form, 157
Vials
    dates on, 64
    explanation of, 5, 23, 27, 136
    multiple-dose, 5, 64, 82–83
    opened by left-handed technicians,
        160
    preparation form for, 157
    reconstituting powdered, 66–67
    single-dose, 23, 27, 64, 136
    use of, 64
    withdrawing from, 65–66
Viruses, linked to cancer, 110
Vitamins, 90
Volume-to-volume (v/v) percentages, 39

W
Weight-to-volume (w/v) percentages, 39
Weight-to-weight (w/w) percentages, 39
Wren, Christopher, 1

Y
Yellow hazardous disposal containers, 113,
    116, 136